If I Should Die Before I Wake

If I Should Die Before I Wake

by

JERRY FALWELL

Thomas Nelson Publishers
Nashville • Camden • New York

Published in Nashville, Tennessee, by Thomas Nelson, Inc., and distributed in Canada by Lawson Falle, Ltd., Cambridge, Ontario.

Printed in the United States of America.

Scripture quotations in this publication are from THE NEW KING JAMES VERSION of the Bible unless otherwise noted. Copyright © 1979, 1980, 1982, Thomas Nelson, Inc.

Scripture references marked KJV are from the King James Version.

Jennifer's last name and a few other names and details have been changed to protect the identities of people involved in this true story.

ISBN 0-8407-5508-2

CONTENTS

If I Should
Die Before
I Wake

Who Will Answer the Challenge?

JERRY

"Dr. Falwell!"

A young newswoman was running along beside me shouting as I walked into the airport terminal building.

"Dr. Falwell," another reporter cried out as my wife, Macel, and I rounded a corner and were confronted by a crowd of news reporters awaiting us there.

Television lights flashed on, almost blinding us by their glare. Television cameras began to record the scene. A battery of microphones was thrust into my face. Flashbulbs popped. Reporters from television and radio stations, newspapers, and newsmagazines had assembled for an extemporaneous press conference in an airport concourse. A large, curious crowd had gathered. On the edge of the crowd a few pickets walked carrying signs. One read, "Abortion, yes! Jerry Falwell, no!"

Almost every place I go, reporters are waiting to question me. For a moment I thought this press conference would be like all the others. I was wrong.

"One more question, please, Dr. Falwell!"

The same young reporter who had run beside me in the terminal was waiting to have her question answered.

"You say that you are against abortion?" she began.

"Yes," I smiled and nodded. Everybody knew exactly how I felt about abortion because I had taken a clear stand against the killing of 1.5 million unborn babies in our country every year. However, this reporter had something else in mind.

"But what practical alternative to abortion do pregnant girls have when they are facing an unwanted pregnancy?" she asked.

"They can have the baby," I answered quickly, too quickly to suit the bright young woman who was questioning me.

"Do you really think it's all that simple?" she asked quietly.

I looked at her for a moment in silence. This was not just a reporter's question, asked to fill space in a paper or on the evening news. The look in the eyes of that reporter made me feel that her question came from deep and private places down inside her.

"Most of the girls in this country facing an unwanted pregnancy are young and poor and helpless," she said, taking advantage of my silence. "They are sometimes victims of incest or are made pregnant by men who misuse and even abuse them. Some are as young as eleven and twelve and thirteen," she continued. "Many of them would be kicked out of their homes, their jobs, their schools the moment their pregnancy even showed. Some would be beaten, their lives threatened by the uncaring and often violent men who made them pregnant or worse yet by their own families."

The young reporter paused. The crowd of reporters waited for my answer.

"What are you doing for women who want to keep their babies but can't find any way to do it?" she asked again. "They have no money for medical treatment let alone to pay for the delivery of their child. They have no way to support themselves, no place to live while they are pregnant. They are young and poor and powerless," she said. "Is it enough to take a stand against abortion," the woman concluded, "when you aren't doing anything to help the pregnant girls who have no other way?"

"No other way," she said, and the words echoed in my mind as the reporters thanked me for the press conference and a policeman led us through the crowd of onlookers who had gathered.

Out of that confrontation a dream was born. I decided that the reporter was right. It wasn't enough to be against abortion. Millions of babies were being killed, and I would go on fighting to save their lives, but what about the other victims of abortion, the mothers of those babies who desperately need help to save their babies?

This book is my answer to that reporter's question. I've asked Jennifer Simpson, one of those courageous young women, to tell her dramatic true story in chapters that alternate with mine. You may know a young lady like her. Or you may be facing this problem now, just as she did. Or you may be simply watching the abortion battle from the sidelines, as I once was, trying to decide what you believe and whether or not to become involved.

"Is there no other way but abortion?"

I believe that we have found an answer to that reporter's question. Read on and see if you agree.

1
Nobody Thought about My Baby

JENNIFER

Finally, the loud metal school bell sounded at the end of my sixth period algebra class. I signed the quiz paper, dropped it on Mrs. Koenig's desk with a sigh, and headed for the door with thirty-two other high school sophomores.

"Thank goodness it's Friday," Shelly Barkman whispered as we walked quickly to our lockers in the hall outside the chemistry lab.

She stopped in front of her locker, whirled the combination back and forth, and finally forced open the bent metal door. I loved to look at the pictures Shelly had taped to the inside of her locker. There was an old black-and-white photo of the Beatles on Abby Road, a shot of Bruce Springsteen in concert holding his guitar in the air, and two pictures of Sting, the lead singer of Police.

But most of Shelly's pictures were photos of her boyfriend, Steve Porter. She had small Polaroid candids of Steve in his varsity football jersey, in his old jeans and a vintage Woodstock T-shirt, and in his Sunday suit and tie. There were pictures of Shelly and Steve together at the junior class dance and at a church youth fellowship beach party on Hartwell Lake. And there was one blowup poster of Steve in his Speedo swimsuit that filled the entire back wall of her locker.

"Look at him," she giggled. "And tomorrow he's mine, all mine."

I wanted to answer that remark with something witty and snide as I left her staring at Steve in his Speedo. But I was too nervous to be nasty. The marble hall echoed with the sounds of boys' voices. I could hear them laughing and yelling and teasing the girls about their weekend plans. I could see them touching and hitting each other playfully and holding hands with their steady girlfriends.

I hardly noticed the girls that year. I thought about boys almost all the time. I could feel them walking by me in the hallway or standing beside me at the lockers or sitting nearby in algebra or world history. Just brushing past a boy going through a classroom doorway made me feel excited and curious and a little afraid.

My locker had no pictures on the door. There was no blowup of a boy in Speedos on the back wall. Those special spaces in my locker were empty and boring, just like my life had been up through my freshman year. But during those last few months as a sophomore, things were changing fast.

"Hi, Jennifer." I looked up quickly into Shelly's boy-friend's blue-blue eyes. "Are you coming with us to the beach?" he asked, putting his books away in the locker next to mine.

"I hope so," I answered. "Mom and Dad are going to a..."

"Good," he yelled over his shoulder heading down the hallway toward Shelly's locker. "See you Saturday."

I stood for a moment looking after him. "Steve is so cute," I remember thinking to myself. "And Shelly is so lucky." There was no boy in my life. Not yet. But during the last few months I felt my luck was changing. During my early teen years I had been a real dog. I tripped over my own feet. My legs were so skinny I wanted to wear long pants to gym class. But my glasses were the very worst thing about me. The lenses were as thick as the bottom of an old Coke bottle. They made my eyes look gigantic, like E.T.'s eyes. Then, when I took my glasses off, my eyes looked tiny and squinty. They blinked every time I tried to focus through the fog. I had felt ugly and rejected and alone most of the time.

"Hi, Jennifer."

It was Mike Erickson and he was speaking to me. Mike was a major item at Jefferson High. I turned slowly to face him. I wanted to say the right thing. I wanted his picture in a racing swimsuit on the back wall of my locker some day.

"Hi, Mike," I said, casually turning back to close my locker and hoping with all my heart that he wouldn't go away.

Mike was already tan from his part-time job as a lifeguard at Ocean Park Swim School. He had curly brown hair and a dimple in his chin. He wore tight faded jeans and a preppy white shirt with the sleeves rolled up past his elbows. His eyes sparkled and his grin made me feel weak and giddy. Every girl I knew had fantasies about Mike and I was no exception. I wanted to turn and take Mike's hand and walk down the hallway with him. Instead, I just stood there with my back to him, fiddling with my locker, hoping he wouldn't walk away and leave me standing alone. Finally, he spoke again.

"Are you going to 'Hart' this weekend?" he asked me.

"Hart" was our nickname for a beach on Hartwell Lake in

Northern Georgia where some of the kids' parents had summer cottages. Shelly's folks had a large house right on the water with a short dock and a ski boat. This early in the season there were long, empty beaches beside the sand dunes and gray gnarled trees and hidden coves with old burned logs from beach parties long past.

"I think so," I answered hopefully. "My parents are going to a conference and said I might be able to spend the weekend with Shelly."

"Terrific," he said, and slapped his hand against the wall above the lockers. "Terrific!"

Then he winked at me and left. I stood there leaning against my locker in total disbelief. Mike was Linda's guy. And Linda was everything I thought that I could never be. She was a cinch to be elected homecoming queen and "The Girl Most Likely to Succeed." With any luck she would be valedictorian and win Miss America on the side. Up against Linda I felt like a real dog again. But Mike had winked at me! Was he a tease? I wondered. Maybe he had something in his eye.

"Stop it, Jennifer," I said to myself, breathing deeply and hoping my heart wouldn't hit 160 beats a minute and kill me off before the weekend. "You aren't a dog anymore, remember? You are a beauty now. At least your dad thinks so. You don't trip over your feet. You aren't skinny. In fact you have great legs, a beautiful body, and contact lenses."

"Mike winked at me," I said again walking quickly from my locker. "Mike winked at me," I whispered to myself as I passed Steve and Mike and two other guys standing around Shelly near her locker.

"We'll be by at 5:30," Shelly yelled when she noticed me. "Be ready."

The guys looked over at me as I passed. They were smiling. Nobody laughed or pointed or whispered something rotten to the others about my skinny legs.

"I'll be ready," I said waving. "Keep your fingers crossed."

Shelly nodded knowingly. My parents were pretty strict. There was a chance they wouldn't let me go.

Then, just that split second before I turned away from the little gang of guys at Shelly's locker, it happened again. Mike winked at me! There was nothing in his eye this time. That moment I knew for certain that I *had* to go on that beach trip whatever my parents thought about it.

I walked as fast as I could toward my home on Jackson Street. My parents had been unable to decide about the weekend at breakfast. They had promised to talk about it during the day and let me know.

"Mike winked at me," I said over and over again as I walked quickly up Pacific Avenue past the 7-11 Market and the Texaco station and down Jackson Street past the library and the bank and the Baptist church where Mom was church secretary and Dad was head deacon.

"Mike winked at me." I was still saying it over and over again as I ran across our lawn, up the cement steps, and through the front door into the living room.

"You're early," Mom said as she came from the kitchen, drying her hands on a dish towel. "Your father isn't home yet."

"Can I go to the beach with Shelly, Mom? Please. It's so important."

She didn't answer right away. She smiled her smile that meant "I've bad news, Daughter," and she sat down beside me on the sofa where I'd flopped.

"Will Shelly's parents be with you at the beach?" she asked.

It wasn't a question. It was an answer. She wanted me to

17

say no so she could explain one more time why it wasn't smart for me to go alone with a group of teenage girls to the beach. But I wanted to go. I don't think I ever wanted anything more in all my life.

Why couldn't she trust me? I thought to myself angrily. I had never really done anything to cause her to doubt me. I was an excellent student. I attended church and Sunday school regularly. I did almost everything that my parents wanted me to do. So, why couldn't my mother trust me, just this one time!

"Mom," I answered trying to keep from shouting at her. "You already know that Shelly's parents aren't going to be there, since they'll be at the same church conference you're going to. But four girls will be there besides Shelly. All their parents have summer cottages near the Barkman's place. We'll be surrounded by parents. Please, Mom," I begged. "You can trust me."

I could tell she wasn't listening. Her head was turned in my direction. Her eyes were looking into mine, but she wasn't listening. She wasn't even trying to understand how important this particular trip was to me and to my future. I had less than one short hour to make her understand.

Please, dear God, I silently prayed. *Make my mother understand.*

"Jennifer," she began and I knew already what was coming. "You know I trust you, but things happen even to trustworthy people if they get themselves into difficult situations."

"Mom, you don't understand. You aren't even trying."

I jumped up from the sofa yelling at her. I knew I should just sit there and talk to her until Dad got home. But I felt crazy and scared. I pictured Mike on that beach with somebody else. I just knew that I would go back to school on Monday and see the two of them together walking through the cafeteria, arm in arm, giggling quietly about their weekend at the beach. And I would be alone again.

"Don't do this to me!" I cried. "You can't!"

Just as I was about to screech something totally hysterical at the top of my lungs, my father walked in.

"That's enough, young lady," he said, walking toward me with his briefcase in one hand and the newspaper in the other. "I won't have you yelling at your mother like that."

My dad hated being caught in the middle between us. But we were both glad when he was there to intervene. Dad was special. Both my parents were, but Dad often took my side in an argument with my mother. After our occasional mother-daughter screamers he would walk me around the block until I cooled down again. Then he would say, "Honey, can't you try to get along with your mother a little better? You know how much she loves you. She's trying her best to do what's right for you. Try to understand her position."

"Understand her position?" I would groan. "Why can't she understand mine?" And so it went. Back and forth. I knew my mother loved me. And I loved her. But during those awkward years, we seemed to be yelling at each other much of the time.

Dad sat us both down at the kitchen table. I apologized for my outburst. Mom made her fears clear to me again. Dad wanted to be sure that the other girls' parents would be nearby, that there would be no drinking, and that there would be no boys at the party. I promised to keep his limits. (I would have promised anything to get out that door and on my way to Hartwell Beach with Shelly and her friends.)

Mom listened quietly. Then she took my hand, swallowed hard, and said that I could go.

I kissed them both, ran to my room, packed jeans, jogging shorts, a sundress, and a bathing suit in a bright red duffle bag and ran back down to say goodbye. Just that moment Shelly and the girls drove into our long driveway.

"You did it," Shelly whispered as we backed slowly down the drive.

"Yes, I did it!" I whispered back loud enough for all the girls to hear.

Marjorie Thomas had made room for me in the front seat. Her parents were divorced, and they lost track of their busy daughter on weekends. Janey Lillas, Ann Blackshaw, Heather Johnston, and Michelle Roberts were crowded into the back seat. Only Heather and Ann still lived with both parents and Ann's dad was an alcoholic. He beat her with a leather belt if she didn't get straight As. Often she came to school with a black eye or bruises on her back or buttocks.

As we drove away, my mother stood on the front porch still holding her dish towel. My dad waved and then walked over to my mom and put his arm around her waist. They both looked sad, as though I was going away forever. Months later my mom told me she had had a terrible feeling about the weekend at the beach, but she didn't want to ruin my fun with her suspicions. I wish now she had.

The day was perfect. The sunset over Hartwell Lake left us quiet and thoughtful. The beach was deserted. Most of the summer places were still empty. We cooked hot dogs over a campfire in Shelly's front yard. We drank Cokes and toasted S'mores and licked the gooey marshmallow and melted chocolate off our fingers.

"Look what I found," Marjorie announced coming down

If I Should Die Before I Wake

from the house carrying two sixpacks of cold beer. Shelly looked panicked for a moment but didn't say anything. The other girls squealed with pretended horror as they rushed to pop open the shiny aluminum cans.

"Drink up, girls," Marjorie ordered lying back onto the sand near the blazing fire. "There's plenty more where this came from."

I didn't drink with them at first. Nobody said a thing about it. When I finally did open a can of my own, it was because I was thirsty and curious and feeling independent. The beer tasted awful at first, but it was cold and bubbly and drinking it made me feel lightheaded and silly. By then everyone was laughing and telling stories on each other and sharing their fantasies about the boys they knew or wished they knew.

At 10:00 P.M. somebody put the last big log on the fire. We were all just lying there staring at the orange and yellow flames when Shelly thought she heard the low growl of Steve's TransAm moving slowly into her driveway. She jumped to her feet and looked into the darkness.

"They've come tonight!" she said, holding her hand over her mouth in pretend surprise.

I stood up also to peer down the driveway at the TransAm coasting toward us, its lights out, its motor silenced. The guys were supposed to come Saturday morning for a day at the beach. That was the promise, but they had changed the plan. The girls groaned and giggled but continued lying around the fire, waiting to be discovered. I jumped up and started away from them down toward the beach. I got up so quickly, I felt dizzy.

"Where are you going?" Shelly whispered.

"I'll be back," I assured her. "I'm just going for a little

walk." My voice sounded husky, and I had difficulty pronouncing the words without slurring them.

"Now?" she asked in disbelief.

"I'll be right back," I answered and hurried into the semi-darkness of the nearby sand dunes. I staggered a little as my feet sank into the sand.

The sky was satin black and laced with stars. I walked as far from Shelly's as I could. I heard a loud honking noise, complete with shouts and whistles, as the guys jumped out to scare the girls who screamed and laughed appropriately. Then all was quiet again. The dunes were just high enough to hide the campfire. I sat on a driftwood log and watched the lake in silence.

I don't really know why I walked away from them that night. It happened very fast. I suppose that I was a little embarrassed. I didn't know who was in the car, but I knew I didn't have a boyfriend coming. I couldn't stand being left out if there were six guys and seven girls. I remembered PE class in junior high school and lining up for teams and never being chosen. I was feeling awkward, too. After all, I was barely sixteen. I didn't have much experience with boys. Also, I admit that I was feeling more than a little bit afraid. On that long ride to the beach the girls had told me what most boys would expect during a romantic night in a beach house on the lake. But I had made a promise, not just a promise to my mom and dad, but a promise to myself. And I was determined to keep it.

"Hi!" Someone spoke out of the darkness. I whirled toward the voice and almost fell from the log. We both laughed as I struggled to regain my balance. It wasn't easy after almost three cans of beer. I felt dizzy and weak and very silly. I was afraid of the "mysterious stranger" but ex-

cited and turned on at the same time. His voice was familiar, but still unknown to me. I never got a good look at his
face.

"Listen to the waves rolling in," he said and I felt his
hands around my waist. For a moment I felt wonderful. To
be held by a boy in the moonlight on a lonely beach was a
dream come true. I had hoped that someone would find me
there. I had even pictured him walking in the dunes calling
my name. I had hoped that he would have blue eyes that
sparkled, and curly brown hair and freckled, suntanned
arms and a grin that would make me feel weak and wonderful. Even in the darkness I expected to see him wink at me.

But when I tried to turn my body toward him to see his
face, his arms gripped me tightly. I couldn't turn. When I
grabbed his arms and tried to push them away, he held me
tighter still. I remember trying to jump off the log, but he
pulled me down and backwards into the sand. I rolled away
from the log and began to crawl towards the top of the
dune. He grabbed my waist and forced my face down into
the sand. The fantasy ended. Suddenly, the romantic dream
became a nightmare.

I don't remember much about what happened next. I
suppose I've pushed it back into some dark corner of my
mind because the memory brings me such awful fear and
anger and sadness. I had dreamed of making love to someone who was in love with me, but that night my dreams
were broken by an act of cruelty and pain and terror.

When he finally disappeared into the darkness, I lay on
my back in the sand staring up at the moon and the stars
and the satin sky, knowing they would never look quite the
same again. Suddenly, I felt that the darkness and the sand
dunes and the quiet sparkling waters were shimmering with

evil. I jumped up and began to run through the dunes down toward the beach and away from the shadows that were pursuing me. My feet sank deep into the sand. I tripped and fell and struggled up again. I couldn't find Shelly's beach house. I don't know how long I ran. I remember a gravel road and sharp rocks cutting my bare feet. I remember seeing the house at last and trying to get my clothes on straight enough to enter and not be noticed. But the lights were off. The beach was empty. The kids were sleeping.

I walked quietly through the boys lying in sleeping bags on the living room floor. I couldn't look down at them. I was afraid I would find him there. Somehow I managed the long flight of stairs and the dark hallway leading to the upstairs bath. I closed the door, locked it, and flooded the room with light. The frightened, frantic face staring back at me from the mirror above the sink was mine. My sundress was ripped at the shoulder. My hair was wet and matted with sand, and my eyes looked wild and afraid. But there was almost no other evidence of the crime. I felt disappointed somehow that there wasn't more to show for what had been done to me.

I remember placing a washrag on the bottom of the tub to kill the sound of hot water running. I remember lying in that tub, scrubbing myself with a washrag but never feeling clean. I remember drying myself and sneaking into the bedroom hoping no one would awaken.

"Jennifer? Is that you?" Shelly whispered sleepily.

"Yeah," I whispered back. "It's me."

"Where've you been?" she asked. "Mike said he didn't see you on the beach."

I climbed into the clean, cold sheets. One of the girls was

snoring. So Mike had been on the dunes. He had looked for me. I couldn't think about it. I wanted to sleep, to forget, to wake up knowing it had never happened.

"Are you O.K.?" Shelly asked in the darkness.

"I'm O.K.," I answered, wanting to scream and to cry and to feel my mother's arms around me.

Somehow I survived the rest of that weekend at the beach and the long drive home. Nobody really questioned my disappearance that night. The girls smiled and looked at me with knowing glances. Of course they were curious. Of course they wanted an explanation. I couldn't give them one even if I tried.

My parents were sitting on the front porch waiting for me when Shelly stopped the car in our driveway. Dad was smiling broadly. Mom just looked relieved. They were happy that their little girl had returned safely from her first big journey into the outside world. It wasn't true. That weekend at the beach would cause our family pain I thought would last forever. From the beginning I knew that awful moment in the dunes would leave me scarred, but I hoped to hide that scar inside me. But something else was growing there that could not be hidden. During that first night at the beach the nagging worry had begun. After three weeks worry changed to panic. In seven weeks I was certain.

"Pregnant?" I asked myself, over and over again. "How could I be pregnant?" I was just sixteen. There was so much I didn't know. I was just a child myself. I couldn't even imagine having one. People had told me that the chances of getting pregnant after being raped were less than 10 percent. Did I prove the statistics wrong? Did they prove I wasn't raped? Whatever happened—and it's still unclear to me because of the foggy memory I have of that night—there was a baby growing inside me and I didn't know what to do about it.

School was over. The summer was hot and sticky and miserable. I was throwing up every morning and tossing and turning throughout each night. I was afraid to tell my parents. I was embarrassed to tell my friends. It seemed too dirty a secret to tell my pastor or my Sunday school teacher. I had never even made an appointment myself with our family doctor or talked to him privately about anything. So I waited. Waiting was my first mistake.

I didn't really understand what it meant to be pregnant. I had seen pictures of a fetus in Mrs. King's health class. But I could hardly picture one growing inside me. And I certainly couldn't think of that fetus as a person. It was something awful that had been left inside me like rubbish that I wanted gone. I was scared all the time. They grew inside me together, the baby and the fear. Finally, I had to tell someone and Shelly seemed the only one who might understand.

"You've got to be kidding," she said when I told her.

"I'm not kidding, Shelly," I replied, desperate for advice.

"What are you going to do?" she asked.

"I thought you could tell me that," I answered.

"Get an abortion," she said immediately. "There's no other way. Girls do it all the time. Ann had one. I think Gracie Stockton did. Other girls keep it secret. I bet lots of our friends have had them and we don't even know about it."

We decided that Mrs. King would know what to do next so I went to school and stopped her outside the office on her way to a summer school class. I felt awkward and rotten and embarrassed.

"You need to see a doctor about an abortion right away," Mrs. King advised as we walked across the campus. "They are quick and harmless," she said. Then she paused and looked at me. "Have you told your parents?"

"Oh, I can't tell them," I stammered. "It would hurt them so much."

Mrs. King interrupted. "Jennifer, if you don't tell them today, I will call and tell them tomorrow." I could tell by the look in her eyes that this was not an idle threat.

At first I was angry that Mrs. King made me tell my parents. Now I am glad. I wish I had told them sooner. I couldn't have hidden my secret much longer anyway, but I had been too miserable and too afraid to do anything before then.

That night at dinner I was trying hard to swallow small bites of chicken and mashed potatoes. Dad and Mom were talking about taxes. I knew the time had come. It was getting hard to breathe. My hands trembled. I forgot the long speech that I had planned and just blurted out the news.

"Mom? Dad? I think I'm pregnant."

My father stopped in midsentence and looked at me in total surprise. My mother stared at me while her eyes filled up with tears. Finally, my dad started asking questions in his quiet, business voice. "Are you sure? How long have you known? Could it be a false alarm?"

We talked almost in whispers back and forth. They asked questions. I answered them. Then my dad grew silent.

"Let's walk," he finally suggested.

We often walked together as a family, especially during times of crisis or tension. That night as we walked my dad asked more questions. My mom cried quietly. I tried to explain.

"How could it have happened?" he said. "Wasn't it a school function? Weren't these kids your friends?"

The more he thought about that beach trip the more he had to struggle to keep his anger in check.

"I'll find that kid," he threatened. "Whoever he is, I'll find him."

We walked and talked for a long time that night. We tried to find a good solution. There was none. Every idea anybody had didn't seem to work. Words flowed back and forth between us. Suggestions were made and dropped again. After a while we ran out of words and walked along in silence. I remember our footsteps echoing on the sidewalk. Although it was early evening and an occasional car drove by, we walked alone on that quiet, tree-lined street. And we were in agony.

"You'll need an abortion." My dad spoke the words slowly as if it hurt to say them. "It's the only option we have. I'll see about it tomorrow."

My mother whispered. "Must we?" she asked him.

My father interrupted her. "Jennifer needs an abortion," Dad repeated. "How can we be idealistic at a time like this?"

We walked back home without saying any more about his decision. Mom went to a nearby drugstore and bought a pregnancy test kit. I filled the little test tube with urine and watched the circle form that proved our fears to be true. Mom stood there in my bathroom staring at the little tube. Then she reached out to hold me and we both began to cry.

In just a few days the decision had been made. Everybody seemed convinced that I needed an abortion: my best friend, Shelly; Mrs. King, my health teacher; my parents. Even Reverend Anderson, a pastor who was a friend of my father's from a nearby town said the Bible says absolutely nothing about "fetal life" and that in my case an abortion seemed a good idea. Everyone agreed that an abortion would be "quick and easy and harmless." In just one brief phone call to a Planned Parenthood office in a town a short drive away the abortion was arranged. Nobody thought about the baby. Not even me.

2

Can We Forget the Little Ones?

JERRY

I will never forget the morning of January 23, 1973. I picked up our newspaper from the front porch of my home in Lynchburg, Virginia, and glanced over it on my way into the kitchen for breakfast. I scanned the headlines telling of Lyndon Johnson's death and for a moment I thought his obituary would be the only newsworthy story of the day. Then I saw the smaller headlines announcing a Supreme Court decision on the controversial matter of abortion.

I don't usually read the paper during breakfast. I glance at the headlines to be sure the world is still in orbit before getting down to the serious business of eggs and bacon and raisin toast. That morning was different. I could not stop reading the story of *Roe* v. *Wade*. The Supreme Court had just made a seven to two decision that would legalize the killing of a generation of unborn children. I couldn't believe that seven justices on that Court could be so callous about the dignity of human life. Were they misinformed? Had they been misled? Were they plunging the nation into

31

a time of darkness and shame without even knowing what they were doing?

My breakfast remained uneaten on my plate. My coffee grew cold as I read and reread the unbelievable story of the Court's decision. I had followed the debate on abortion with growing interest. I had read articles by Dr. Francis Schaeffer and Dr. Jack Willke discussing the implications for a society that condones the mass killings of its unborn children. I had talked to doctors and social workers about the physical and psychological effects on the women who choose abortion to end an unwanted pregnancy. I had preached on abortion and its meaning to my people and had used abortion as an example in several sermons over the past ten years. But, as I read the paper that day, I knew something more had to be done, and I felt a growing conviction that I would have to take my stand among the people who were doing it.

I knew immediately that the nation would be painfully divided by this issue. President Nixon had just been sworn into his second term of office by Chief Justice Burger. The president was against abortion, but the chief justice had sided with the pro-abortion majority of the Court. The church, too, would be divided with the pro-life opposition led by the Roman Catholic Church.

"How many millions of children prior to their birth will never live to see the light of day because of the shocking action of the majority of the United States Supreme Court today?" asked New York's Terence Cardinal Cook.[1]

"It is hard to think of any decision in the two hundred years of our history which has had more disastrous implications for our stability as a civilized society," warned John Joseph Cardinal Krol, the president of the National Conference of Catholic Bishops.[2]

I felt confident that most traditionally conservative churchmen, lay and clergy alike, would agree with the Catholics, while most traditionally liberal churchmen, lay and clergy alike, would applaud the court's decision on behalf of the rights of pregnant women.

Immediately, response began to flow into the Supreme Court building from around the country. Court guards had to set up large bins in the basement to sort the letters, telegrams, and petitions to each justice condemning the Court's decision. Those who saw the letters remember critics comparing the justices "to the butchers of Dachau, to child killers, to immoral beasts, and to Communists."[3] Some people even threatened the justices' lives or sent letter bombs to the Supreme Court Building. Hysteria, I knew, would not bring meaningful or lasting change; rash words and actions would only dishonor the cause. But something had to be said to save the millions of unborn children who would die. Something had to be done on their behalf.

Again I began to preach against abortion, sincerely hoping that words would be enough. I called abortion "America's national sin." I compared abortion to Hitler's "final solution" for the Jews and the Court's decision to setting loose a "biological holocaust" on our nation. Almost immediately I knew in my heart that preaching would not be enough. Opponents of the Court's decision were taking their protest to the streets. For the first time in my life I wanted to be there with them, taking my stand on behalf of this life-and-death issue.

But becoming politically active was not easy for this Baptist preacher. I had always tried to be a responsible citizen in the privacy of the voting booth. My school teachers had taught me the concept of the separation of church and state and I had faithfully practiced that belief. In fact, during the

1960s when liberal churchmen were marching in front lines for every cause imaginable, I had been stunned and appalled by their behavior. In 1965 I preached a sermon entitled "Ministers and Marches." In that sermon I expressed my honest feelings that "government could be trusted to correct its own ills." People were descending on Washington by the hundreds of thousands to march for every kind of issue from legalizing marijuana to ending the war in Vietnam. Some of the issues I favored. Others I opposed. However, I believed then that the Christian's best contribution to social change was his or her faithfulness to our primary goals: studying the Word, preaching the gospel, winning souls, building churches and Christian schools, and praying for the eventual healing of the nation.

At ministers' meetings I had preached against the clergy's taking an active role in political causes. Again, I told my fellow pastors across the country that they could trust government to correct itself. "Our role as pastors and Christian leaders," I had said, "is to attend to the spiritual needs of our people." Serving the church and letting government take care of itself had been my lifelong policy.

I had begun the Thomas Road Baptist Church in Lynchburg, Virginia, in 1956, when I was only twenty-two years old. We started our little church with thirty-five members, and I had done almost nothing else but serve that growing congregation for seventeen years. Practically, there hadn't been time to do anything else. Over the years, our Christian education ministry had expanded to include an academy, a college, and a program of continuing education for thousands of students. Our evangelism program had grown to include a worldwide television and radio ministry, along with the publication of books, pamphlets, and study guides. By the time of the *Roe* v. *Wade* decision, I was preacher, teacher, chief executive officer, and pastor to a congregation of over fifteen thousand members. At first I was convinced that there was no time in the day to do more than preach or teach against abortion and pray that someone else would risk his life and vocation on behalf of millions of unborn babies whose lives were in jeopardy.

Also, I reminded myself, when fundamentalist Christians finally get involved in political issues, they often betray their own ignorance about the problems and their naivete about the political processes that lead to solutions. This Supreme Court decision was no exception. In the immediate outpouring of public sentiment against the legalization of abortion, more than one thousand Baptists and similar religious groups sent angry letters and telegrams to Justice Hugo Black condemning his participation in the Court's decision. Justice Black had been dead for sixteen months. The writers of those letters had their hearts in the right place but they were uninformed and thus ineffective. If I were to become involved, I knew I would have to understand the legal process and the complex issues. There would be books and pamphlets and legal briefs to read. There would be experts and authorities to interview.

There was another good reason to stay away from the complex and explosive abortion issue. I believed in a pluralistic nation. I pastored a church where people could hold various political views and still be one in Christ. Already the nation was being divided over the issue. Would that also happen to my congregation?

There were plenty of reasons to let this issue pass, but the more I thought about the killing of the unborn child, the more I knew my reasons were not reasons at all, but excuses, excuses to save me from the extra work, from the risk, from the pressures and the embarrassment of taking a stand in an arena where I had not taken a stand before.

One day not long after the Supreme Court's decision, I saw a full-color picture of an unborn child approximately sixteen to eighteen weeks old. The child's eyes were closed. She was sound asleep, sucking her thumb, floating in a silken sack, waiting for that moment when she would decide that her time inside had ended and her time outside would begin. She had delicate, graceful fingers and toes. Her skin was shiny and transparent. You could see her vital organs shadowed in shades of pink and red. Her heart, already beating 120 to 160 times a minute, was pumping blood that she herself had made to her perfectly shaped arms and legs and torso and then back through her heart again through a weblike maze of microscopic veins.

In that picture I saw a tiny, trusting child whom God had created. Regardless of the human reasons behind this child's conception, God loved her. It didn't matter if her human parents wanted her to live or die. God wanted her to live. The Supreme Court of the United States of America had made a terrible mistake. Because of their decision that tiny, unborn miracle of God's creation could be killed with the consent of her mother, the medical profession, and the highest court of the land. Now I was certain my position was valid, but I still hesitated to take a public stand.

It was my family who finally helped me decide to become active in the pro-life movement. During the winter of 1974, almost a year after the Supreme Court's decision, we were sitting around a roaring fireplace in the living room of our home in Lynchburg. My older son, twelve-year-old Jerry, had just read a passage from the book of Revelation describing the final return of Christ to earth. My ten-year-old daughter, Jeannie, sat in my wife's lap. And my youngest son, Jonathan, an eight-year-old redhead, was lying on the floor looking up at me.

During the course of that night's family altar time I shared, a bit too freely, my own skepticism regarding our nation's health. I must have been tired that night for I said dark, gloomy things about the future. Frankly, I was concerned, perhaps more than I ever had been before. The country had so deteriorated during that last decade that I feared for my children's future. I honestly believed that what my wife and I had known of the greatness and the goodness of this country, our children might never know.

The laundry list of America's ills was long and disheartening. While abortion was at the top of my list of priorities that needed attention, there were others: pornography, drugs, the 40 percent divorce rate, sex without commitment, children without marriage, and the growing hostility of our young people toward the family, the church, free enterprise, and the nation. The country seemed doomed. The trends toward liberalism and hedonism seemed irreversible. We were entering a new age of secular humanism, and I was afraid for my country and for my children who were growing up just as my country seemed to be falling apart.

Throughout my tired-father confession that night I used the legal murder of millions of America's unborn children as a primary example of the terrible condition in which the country found itself.

"Why don't you do something about it, Dad?" my spunky red-headed son finally interrupted, rising up on one elbow and looking me in the eye.

"Yeah," chimed in my daughter. "Do something for the babies."

I tried to explain to them that there was little I could do.

We lived in a small town in the Blue Ridge Mountains of Virginia. We had no great financial resources. We had no political power or influence on people with that power. I was already working twenty-five hour days even though I wanted to spend more time with my family. I made a list of excuses that silenced but did not seem to convince them.

Twenty-four hours passed. The next night the three children came to our family altar prepared to blast my excuses out of the water. Apparently they had been thinking about my words. They didn't want to face a bleak, frightening future. They told me in no uncertain terms that it was my responsibility as their father to get off my chair and go out into the world and do what I could to make a difference.

"Dad, you know those babies you were talking about last night" said my twelve year old, "those babies that are getting killed? You ought to try to stop it."

My children hounded me those next few weeks. They never stopped reminding me about the babies who were dying. I began to pray and think seriously about this task and the others. Honestly, I didn't have the foggiest idea what I as one insignificant Baptist preacher in Lynchburg, Virginia, could do to influence a nation. But as I thought and prayed and argued with my own kids, convictions began to grow. My nation had made some wrong choices. At the top of the list was the legalization of abortion. What would they legalize next? The killing of the handicapped? The killing of the aged? The killing of the ill? Something needed to be done. There was only one way I knew to do it, and I could delay that task no longer.

One day I was a Baptist preacher who had managed to stay out of the political arena for twenty years of ministry. The next day I jumped into that same political arena feet first. At the heart of my decision was a story from the New

Testament. Jesus' enemies, the Pharisees, had gathered to trick and trap Him in a public debate.

"Is it lawful to pay taxes to Caesar, or not?" the Pharisees asked, looking around at the crowd, knowing that either way Jesus answered He would be in trouble. If He answered, "No, don't pay taxes to the government," the soldiers would arrest Him and throw Him in jail. If He answered, "Yes, pay your taxes," He would offend the people who hated the government and wanted to see it overthrown. Jesus didn't answer immediately. Instead, He called for a Pharisee to hold up a coin used in paying the tax.

"Whose image and inscription is this?" Jesus asked.

"Caesar's," answered the Pharisees.

"Then render to Caesar the things that are Caesar's and to God the things that are God's."

It was a clever answer. Both sides were satisfied. But it wasn't only clever. Jesus' answer cut to the heart of our human predicament. We live in two different worlds simultaneously. The world that God is building in the hearts of men and women is an invisible world based on eternal values that will last forever. The world that man is building is a world of cement and steel and glass based on human values that will not last. The trouble is that we live in both worlds simultaneously. We who are committed to the invisible world of God and to His values cannot simply stand aside while the other world destroys itself and the world we share. In that confrontation with the Pharisees, Jesus reminded us that though our first allegiance is to God and His goals for this planet, we must still be responsible citizens, willing to play our part in maintaining the world of man.

There was a second important reminder for me in that

story. When Jesus said, "Render to Caesar the things that are Caesar's, and to God the things that are God's," He was not just telling us to be responsible in both worlds, He was also reminding us to keep the worlds apart. Each world works differently. What we do in God's world and with His people has different rules from what we do in the world of government with elected officials and volunteers. America is not a theocracy, a government with God as its commander-in-chief. America is a democratic republic with a man (perhaps one day, a woman) as its chief executive officer. In God's world, we decide by God's rules. In a democratic republic, we work together, governed by the will of the majority. In God's world, we submit to Him. In man's world we submit to the law of man.

But a third, unwritten truth of this story, which Jesus made clear by His life and by His death, kept me from ignoring the Supreme Court's decision. Although we live in two worlds simultaneously and although both worlds are to be kept separate, when there is a conflict between the worlds, the world of God takes precedence over the world of man. When we feel the law of man is unjust or contrary to the law of God, we work to change man's law. And if the law of man actually comes into conflict with the law of God, we disobey man's law and pay the penalty.

We cannot forget God's law as we live in man's world. We must live by God's law in both worlds, whatever it may cost us. We must work to convince others that God's law is right and will bring health and long life to the nation. We do not insist on others' believing as we believe, or worshiping as we worship. We protect the freedom of every person in the land. But if we feel a law is wrong or harmful for the nation, we work tirelessly to change it. And we use every legal tool to accomplish that end.

During my first years of ministry, I had given to God what was God's and had almost eliminated my responsibility to Caesar (government) altogether. I had paid my taxes, of course. I had voted. I had occasionally made a call or written a letter or carried on a conversation to influence public policy. From time to time my sermons commented on issues of significance to the nation. But to work hard to change public policy or to dedicate time and energy to influence government was a new experience for me. I had spent my lifetime working in the context of the church, God's world. I knew how to bring change in that world, but to bring change to the world of city, state, and national government was new.

It didn't happen overnight. First, I began to read everything I could get my hands on concerning the issues that were high on my priority list. My reading habits had been fairly limited to the Bible, biblical reference books, commentaries, church history, ethics, theology, psychology, and philosophy. There were books, journals, magazines, and articles that helped me in sermon preparation and in the development of my spiritual life. To round out the other side, the secular side, I had just read the newspaper and various newsmagazines. I had watched television news, public broadcasting, and various documentaries on the subjects of special interest to me and to my people at the Thomas Road Baptist Church.

Once I entered the political arena, I realized my study habits would have to be enlarged. The news magazines gave short, encapsulated, often one-sided reviews of current events. I had to read papers, journals, and special reports that gave fuller, deeper coverage. I began to read both sides of the complex abortion issue. I read the *Congressional Record*, medical and scientific studies, journals of the pro-life and pro-choice groups, summaries of the court decisions, and papers, books, and articles from many points of view.

I traced the Supreme Court's decision back to the beginning of the legal battle. I learned that early in 1971, a young woman in Texas, not unlike our own Jennifer, found herself pregnant and wanted to abort her child. The laws of the state of Texas said, "No! Although we respect your right of choice, we are also committed to protecting the rights of the unborn child living within you." In Texas, as in a majority of states, abortion was illegal unless the mother's life was threatened. The young woman, named "Jane Roe" by the United States District Court for the Northern District of Texas, sued the state to have the law revoked. The court decided in Jane Roe's favor.

According to the court, Jane Roe's right to choose whether to have a child or to abort it was "protected by the 9th through the 14th Amendments of the U.S. Constitution." The federal court declared that the Texas laws against abortion were void because they were "unconstitutionally vague and overbroad." Texas appealed the court's decision to the United States Court of Appeals for the Fifth Circuit. Eventually, the case was heard by the United States Supreme Court.

The abortion issue was a hot potato thrown back and forth by the nine justices for more than two years between the opening arguments heard December 13, 1971, and the Court's final decision, January 22, 1973. Chief Justice Burger assigned Justice Blackmun, a fellow Minnesotan, the difficult task of writing the majority opinion. The justices, their clerks, and secretaries prepared memo after memo, rough draft after rough draft, trying to reach a conclusion that would properly interpret the Constitution on this important matter.

But the Constitution itself provided no specific guidelines on the abortion issue. The 14th Amendment to the United States Constitution had been quoted in Jane Roe's trial by her lawyers to protect the young woman's right to abort her baby. But it was also quoted by lawyers for the state of Texas to protect Jane Roe's unborn child from abortion. The 14th Amendment states simply:

Nor shall any state deprive any person of life, liberty or property without due process of law, nor deny to any person within its jurisdiction the equal protection of the laws.

Both sides, those who favor the legalization of abortion (sometimes called "pro-choice") and those who oppose abortion (sometimes called "pro-life") quote the 14th Amendment when making their cases. However, in 1868 when the 14th Amendment was adopted, at least thirty-six states or territories had laws on the books limiting abortion. Those anti-abortion laws were not changed when the 14th Amendment was ratified, making it clear that the framers of the 14th Amendment did not originally intend to use it to keep the states from regulating abortions.

As Justices Rehnquist and White pointed out later in their dissenting opinions, nothing in the language or history of the Constitution supported the Court's judgment to legalize abortion. Justice Blackmun, formerly a legal advisor to the Mayo Clinic in Rochester, Minnesota, turned to medical and social policy, not to the law, to guide him in writing the Court's decision. Wearing a cardigan sweater and working at an isolated mahogany table hidden in the second floor library of the Supreme Court Building, Justice Blackmun read hundreds of legal briefs, medical books, and memos from his fellow justices and their clerks in his honest struggle to do justice to the millions of people born and unborn who would be affected by the Court's decision. His clerks, secretaries, and messengers were warned not to interrupt the justice as he puzzled over the complex and confounding materials. Even Chief Justice Burger and the other seven justices of the Court knew not to bother him there.

Justice Blackmun decided that his major responsibility was to protect the rights of choice and privacy of the pregnant woman guaranteed her by the United States Constitution. Here, medical science misled the Court in advising the justices that the fetus was not a person and had no rights to be protected, at least not in the first three months after conception. During the first trimester, the fetus was seen as tissue, a nonperson without Constitutional rights or privileges. Most medical authorities saw the unborn child as "not very much a person" up through the second three months of pregnancy. Many medical experts even claimed the fetus was a nonperson through the entire pregnancy. To these authorities, the fetus only became a "viable" person when delivered out of the mother and into the world, free from the mother's life support systems and able to survive on its own.

If Justice Blackmun had regarded the fetus as a person, then that person, though unborn, would be protected by the Constitution. He did not. But to avoid the controversy he knew would follow, the justice left out any direct discussion of the viability of the fetus and tried to dodge the issue in a complex discussion of the three trimesters of pregnancy. However, before Justice Stewart would add his signature to the majority decision, he insisted that Justice Blackmun say more clearly that a fetus wasn't a person. Justice Blackmun consented to his colleague's request. "A fetus," wrote Justice Blackmun, "is not a person under the Constitution and thus has no legal right to life."

During the first three months of pregnancy, the Supreme Court instructed the courts in every state that, "the abortion decision and its effectuation must be left to the medical judgment of the pregnant woman's attending physician." After the first trimester, a state may "regulate the abortion procedure in ways that are reasonably related to maternal health," for example, by requiring hospitalization. Only after the fetus has developed enough to have a chance of survival on its own—usually during the seventh month—may a state "regulate and even proscribe abortion except where it is necessary...for the preservation or health of the mother."[4]

The state of Texas, after losing its appeal, petitioned for rehearing, comparing Blackmun's decision (that a fetus was not a person) to the Court's decision in 1857, which stated that Dred Scott, a black slave, was not a citizen or person under the Constitution.[5]

Once I understood the judicial history of the abortion decision, I began to study government and how it works. I learned that the wall of separation that my school teachers had said divided church and state was not even mentioned in the United States Constitution. In fact, the words *church* and *state* were not part of the First Amendment, as some people suggested. Thomas Jefferson wrote these words in a letter in 1802 to a group of Baptists and Congregationalists in Danbury, Connecticut. During Jefferson's campaign for president, the group attacked him, calling him an infidel, an atheist, and a few other uncomplimentary names.

Jefferson told them they should stay in their place. There should be "a wall of separation between church and state," he had said. The principle I had been taught so long ago was not a part of the Constitution, as I had always believed.

I also learned the principles of changing and affecting government policies. There were babies to be saved and in order to save them I had to learn about voter registration, district door-to-door campaigning, legislative lobbying, and power politics. My library looked like a battle zone. Every room in our home was loaded with reading materials. I kept notes on the important findings in my study. I copied quotations that were meaningful or carried emotional clout. In my brain a plan was beginning to take shape.

Next, I began to associate with people who knew about the issues and who could help me understand them better, even if I didn't agree with them. I began to make regular calls to congressmen and senators. I called and telegraphed and visited with leaders on the abortion issue from around the country. I visited pro-life group meetings and talked to pro-life leaders. I visited pro-choice groups and talked to their leaders as well. I met Christians, Jews, Moslems, agnostics, and atheists who were all Americans and who all had something to teach me about the issue. I listened. I talked. I argued. And I learned.

Already, critics were condemning me for entering the political world. They were even quoting my old sermon from 1965, "Ministers and Marches," in which I had clearly called pastors away from what I was now doing. I received nasty letters and telegrams from Christian friends and allies chastising me for associating with "worldy people," warning me to get out of politics and back into religion where I belonged. And from a third and more frightening group, hidden behind unsigned letters and mysterious phone calls in the night, I began to get ugly threats against my life and the lives of my family. But I had committed myself to helping save the babies and their mothers, both victims of the Court's decision on abortion, and there was no turning back.

Whatever small risks we take to save a Jennifer and her baby are worth it; Jennifer is only one example of the millions of young women who have recently chosen to abort their unwanted babies. As she shares with us her own private memories of the abortionist and his clinic, try to feel how she felt that awful day her baby died.

3

Take Two Cookies and a Glass of Milk

JENNIFER

The Sunday morning paper hit our driveway with a loud thud. I opened my eyes and stared for a moment at the ceiling. Whatever dream I had been dreaming was gone. I couldn't bring it back. Then I heard music in the kitchen. Mom was listening to a church choir on the radio. The smell of bacon sizzling in the iron skillet usually brought back memories of happy Sunday mornings in my childhood. That day the smell of bacon made me sick. I could feel my stomach churning, and I wanted to ignore it. I closed my eyes and tried to sleep again, but I could not escape my daily bout of morning sickness. Unwillingly, I stumbled from my bed, ran to the bathroom, and sent signals to my family that another day of pregnancy had begun.

Even as I stood staring into those whirling waters I remembered: This would be the last day of my pregnancy. I was going to have an abortion. Abortion. The word was ugly to me then and it is uglier to me now. During those last few days everyone convinced me that an abortion during

49

the first twelve weeks of pregnancy was "no big deal." Mrs. King had said that abortion is "a regular procedure with nothing to worry about." My friend Shelly smiled and assured me that "all our friends are having one." *Relax,* I told myself. *You're only having an abortion.*

As I showered that special Sunday morning I felt tremendous relief. The warm water splashed on my face and ran down my body. I scrubbed my arms and legs with soap and watched the lather drain away. Whatever he had left in me would soon be gone forever. After the abortion I would be clean again.

"Jennifer? Are you all right?" My mother stood at the door of my bathroom and called out to me.

"I'm fine, Mom. I'll be right down," I replied.

I was glad Mom and Dad were both going to drive me to Richmond, a small community just sixty miles from our home. We would be gone for only half a day. The Planned Parenthood people had promised that the abortion would take only four hours or less. "There will be slight discomfort and appropriate inconvenience," the social worker told us on the phone, "but in a few short days you will be as good as new again."

"Good morning, Jen," my father said putting down the Sunday paper as I walked into the kitchen. "How's my girl?"

I didn't know how to tell either of my parents how much I needed them. It was such a relief that they were going to stand by me. That morning no one even spoke the word. No one blamed me. No one made me feel guilty. No one even cried. We were a family and what we had to face we would face together.

Don't misunderstand. We had argued and fought and cried a lot. We would argue and fight and cry again. We all had our down times when the shock of my pregnancy and the problems it created got to us. Each of us had said things we wished we hadn't said, and each of us had had to say, "I'm sorry." Through it all my parents were on my side and I knew that they were with me even in the bad times.

"It's time," my dad announced and pushed his chair away from our breakfast table. "I'll call to confirm our appointment. You two get ready. We don't want to be late."

Suddenly, my mother looked quite pale. I didn't know until then how much she had struggled over the abortion decision. She started to get up from the table and then sat back down again.

"Are you OK, Mom?" I asked moving around to sit beside her.

"I'm fine," she said looking up at me. "I'm just feeling very sad."

I sat beside her, watching her struggle against the tears. Mom had eight miscarriages before having a little girl. Losing those eight unborn children was devastating for both of them. When my mother finally went nine months, the baby girl was born with a congenital heart defect. Little baby Emily was in and out of the hospital for months. Then, when she was only nine months old, her heart stopped beating in the middle of the surgery necessary to repair it.

Now I look back on that Sunday morning of my abortion and know better the pain and sadness my mother must have felt that day.

"I really am fine," she said again, placing her hand on mine. "And how are you?"

I smiled. "I feel OK, Mom! In just a few hours it will all be over," I said, hoping that it would be true. I didn't believe it then. I don't believe it now. They lie who tell you that an abortion is "harmless." They lie who say an abortion is "quick and painless." They lie who lead you to believe that "in just a few hours it will be all over." There are some things we never really get over. To say we do is to tell a lie. Still, that Sunday morning of my abortion I felt relief because I believed the lie then.

On the twelve-block drive to the freeway from our home we passed First Church. The parking lot was filling rapidly with friends and neighbors we had known for years. No one noticed us drive by. I suppose we didn't want them to notice. And yet, for almost every Sunday of my life my family and I had driven slowly into that church parking lot together. We had walked into the sanctuary together. We had sat together through the singing of the hymns and the praying of the prayers and the preaching of the sermon. We had attended Sunday school classes there and potluck suppers and youth meetings and deacon meetings and prayer and Bible study meetings. It still makes me sad to think that on the Sunday of my abortion nobody even looked up as we drove by.

The morning was gray and overcast. Thunderclouds were forming over the city. The wind was beginning to shake the flowered bushes that line the freeway divider. Junk was blowing across the four-lane road. Dirty paper plates and empty beer cans, leaves and crumpled cardboard cartons soon littered the highway. The car bumped and weaved in the wind just enough to make me ill. Two times we had to stop for bouts of morning sickness. Each time that we stopped, my dad grew more nervous about the time. I got defensive. My mother grew quieter.

By the time we arrived at the clinic, we were irritable and

grumpy with each other. In fact, it wasn't the ride or the wind or the littered highway or the bouts of morning sickness that plagued us. It was the unknown that made us scared—the growing concern if what we were doing was right. It was the intuition that underneath this easy answer were questions we hadn't asked or answered at all.

Dad parked at the curb in front of a one-story medical center with a small gold Planned Parenthood sign in the corner window. There were at least half a dozen other cars in the parking lot nearby. We walked together toward that place pretending it was just another family chore. We wanted to believe that this was like going to the dentist to have a bad tooth removed or to a dermatologist to have a harmless growth burned away.

When we entered the clinic, a receptionist slid open a glass window and leaned forward to greet us. "Can I help you?" she asked.

"Jennifer Simpson has an appointment at eleven o'clock," my dad responded.

The woman looked down at her appointment book and smiled at me. "Please be comfortable," she said gesturing toward a sofa. "We'll call you in a few minutes."

After an eternity of silence, a nurse entered the reception area. "Please follow me, Jennifer," she said smiling. "We'll be ready for you right away."

Mom reached out to touch me as I left, and my dad just stood there looking awkward. They weren't alone. The room was filled with dads and moms and boyfriends. They all had that same unsmiling, waiting-room look on their faces. They were all staring at pictures in old magazines they didn't see and were turning pages they didn't read.

I was glad to leave them and followed the nurse into a small office where she handed me one of those horrible hospital gowns with no back and practically no front and strings you can't reach to tie and once they're tied you can't untie them to save your life.

"Will you fill this please?" she said handing me an empty bottle. I filled it. They checked it. They told me what I knew already. I was pregnant.

But while I waited for the test results, I sat in an inner conferencelike room filled with other girls with unwanted pregnancies. We sat in a circle facing each other. At first no one spoke. They also were teenagers. Two appeared to be thirteen or fourteen; two others were seventeen or eighteen. One was my age.

At first we looked around the room trying not to see each other but stealing occasional glances, reading the unspoken words written in each other's eyes. One by one the girls began to cry. First, they sniffled. Lips trembled. Eyes grew damp. Fingers gripped the paper gowns and tried to make them cover. Then the tears began to flow, followed by real sobs and coughs and body-shaking sighs.

I thought to myself, *What in the world am I doing here?* It was a small room filled with crazy, crying girls. Somebody had to get control. Somebody had to say something, and I was the only somebody not in tears.

"Hi," I said quietly. "My name is Jennifer."

"I'm Lauralee," the thirteen year old answered immediately. "And I'm scared to death."

That confession was all it took.

"We're all scared to death!" we answered in unison. And before long everybody was laughing and talking about their boyfriends and remembering the times they had been in that room.

"You've been here before?" I asked the fourteen year old, trying not to show my surprise.

"Yeah," she said quietly. "Just three months ago."

"Me, too," said the seventeen year old. "Twice."

"Twice?" I said, looking more surprised than ever.

"Jeannie and I have been here twice," the older girl said. "And one time I did it in L.A. on a vacation."

A nurse entered the room. The girls grew silent.

"Good morning, girls," she said cheerily. "I know some of you don't need to hear my little speech, but for you new-comers this information is important."

Then she began a rather thorough discussion of the abortion procedures and of recommended follow-up care upon our return home. The girls listened sleepily. One even dozed. I thought of the airline stewardess's message at the beginning of a flight. The stewardess talks about the possibilities of surviving an air crash and nobody even listens. I listened to that nurse, but what she said didn't make sense to me. So, like all the others, I finally tuned her out.

"Jennifer Simpson?" The nurse had finished her lecture and asked me to follow her from the room. I suppose we didn't really listen to the nurse for the same reason passengers on an airplane don't really listen to the warnings of a stewardess. Who wants to hear bad news? Who wants to know what we should do about it? We turn our safety over to the stewardesses or the doctors and the nurses and hope they will take care of us. And we never really learn to take care of ourselves. So, when the plane does crash and explode into flames on the runway, nobody knows what to do. The passengers die clutching in their hands the emergency instructions they did not bother to listen to or to read.

"It can't happen to me," I said the first time, but it did. "It certainly can't happen to me the second time," I said as I listened to the girls in the room that day, but I would be wrong again.

"Lie down on the table, please, Jennifer," the nurse instructed me. "And we'll have you out of here in no time."

The shiny metal table was covered with paper like the paper I was wearing. I lay my head back against a pillow in a paper pillow case and lifted my legs into the stirrups high above me.

"The doctor will be right in," the nurse added, swabbing my left forearm with some kind of cleansing solution. "Just try to relax and think about something pleasant," she counseled me as she rushed out the door to handle one of the other girls in a room like mine.

I'll always remember how embarrassed I felt that day when the young male doctor entered the room to find my two bare legs sticking almost straight into the air and my hands gripping the table for dear life.

"Hello, Jennifer," he said. "Everything will be fine." He called for the nurse, who returned immediately and handed the doctor a round metal tube that looked sharp on one end and hollow. I later learned this was the suction tube.

"This will hurt a little," he said, as he inserted a needle into the back of my hand.

It hurt a lot. In fact I gripped the table with my free hand and pressed hard against the table.

No, no, no, I cried to myself. *It can't hurt this bad. It can't.*

"And you may taste a slight bit of garlic as it takes effect," the doctor continued calmly.

It tasted awful. I haven't been able to eat garlic since that day. When I get really depressed or sick, I taste the garlic all over again. Even an Italian restaurant or a pizza parlor makes me remember the shock and the sadness.

The anesthesia began to take effect.

I don't know what he did to me after that.

I woke up on a bed. A nurse was removing a bloody pad from between my legs. It was gross. I'll never forget it. I didn't know that you could bleed so much and still survive. I lay there thinking I was going to die when the receptionist entered the room and placed a glass of milk and a plate of Oreo cookies beside me.

"How 'bout a little snack," she said, "before you head home?"

I looked at those two cookies and the glass of milk and I felt terribly foolish. It didn't look anything like a last supper. The abortion was over. I was fine. I remembered very little pain. The intruder was gone forever. I felt weak and dizzy and high.

"How are you feeling, Jennifer?" the young doctor asked as he hurried into the room between patients.

"Fine," I answered. "No problem."

"Jennifer," he said, "there is a way to keep this from happening again."

I nodded hoping that would be enough to get him out of there so I could get into my clothes and be back with my folks again.

"This package contains a month's supply of birth control pills," he said, holding up a circular package with round, pink pills in tiny, punch-out pockets.

"Take them," he ordered. "The package tells you when and being here today should tell you why." He held the pills out to me. I didn't want to take them. Embarrassed and angry at the same time, I knew another way to keep it from happening again. I didn't like what he was suggesting. I didn't need pills to keep me off that table with my feet up in stirrups and my bare legs sticking out of a worthless paper gown. But he stood there holding them out to me. Finally, I took the pills.

"Thanks," I said meekly, hoping he would go away.

"Now, eat your cookies," he said with a smile. "The nurse will help you into your clothes and you can join your dad and mom."

Closing the door quietly he left me alone on that table with the cookies and milk and the birth control pills. I put the pills down on the table beside me. As I ate the cookies and drank the milk I tried to figure out how I could hide the pills from Mom and Dad. I hid them in my purse, determined to flush them down the nearest toilet. Then, with a quick sugar rush from the Oreos, I dragged myself into my clothes and out to the room where my mom and dad were waiting.

"How do you feel, Jen?" my father asked taking one arm while my mother took the other.

"I'm fine, Dad," I answered quickly. "Really, it was nothing."

Actually I was still bleeding slightly and I would bleed for another two or three weeks before I healed completely. My muscles were tight and sore. It hurt to walk, but I didn't really need assistance. It just felt good to have my parents there, one on either side, helping me.

We walked back through the reception room. Other families were waiting for the girls inside. New girls and their folks were entering the clinic or parking in the lot outside. There was a steady stream of girls just like me who were led to that place for their abortions. I wonder now, as I look back, if they knew as little as I had known about what would really happen there.

4

When Does the Miracle Begin?

JERRY

In a quiet, tree-lined grotto on Liberty Mountain there is a monument to Jennifer's baby and to millions of other babies killed by abortion. Surrounded by a natural rock wall and gardens alive with flowers, the marker reads: "In memory of the millions of aborted babies that have died in America since January 22, 1973."

A Scripture reference is included at the base of the memorial: "But whoso shall offend one of these little ones…, it were better for him that a millstone were hanged about his neck, and that he were drowned in the depth of the sea" (Matt. 18:6).

The words carved into that giant marble tombstone are the only memorial I know to the one and a half million babies aborted in this country on an average every year. Their tiny bodies—or the fragments that remain—are not even given the rights of burial. Every day new horror stories about infant remains are reported by the media.

The motion picture *Conceived in Liberty* (distributed by

American Portrait Films) documents one of many such stories from a suburb of Los Angeles. A large dumpster, discovered in the back yard of a medical pathologist's home, was stuffed wall to wall, floor to ceiling, with the remains of seventeen thousand human babies.

The supervisor tells how he first heard about the dreadful contents of that dumpster. "I got a radio call from Ron Gillette, the foreman. He said the men were throwing up, and there was something wrong."

What would cause those rugged crew members to vomit?

Here is their own description of that day, taken directly from the filmed interviews:

"One of them fell down and hit me right in front of my feet. And there it was," one man remembered. It was a mutilated body....And the closer I looked at it, it was a human body."

Another man continued. "I couldn't believe it. Little bitty babies all torn to pieces. Hands chopped off, arms, legs. Just makes you sick to see something like that....Well, really it makes you want to cry when you see something like that."

"I really don't want to witness it again," said still another man. "Not what I saw."

When city officials were notified, forty-four of the tiny corpses were autopsied. The babies had been aborted after nineteen to twenty-seven weeks of life. They showed evidence of every possible abortion technique. Some of the bodies were whole but blackened or stained by chemical abortions. Most of the bodies were mutilated or broken into pieces by abortionist tools. Apparently the bodies had been obtained by the pathologist to use in scientific experiments after their abortions.

When Does the Miracle Begin?

"In early November 1982," another typical abortion story begins, "a workman at a Wichita, Kansas, incinerator was burning bags of unidentified 'pathological waste' from Wesley Medical Center in Wichita, when he discovered that one of the bags contained bodies of dead babies. Horrified, the worker notified authorities and then called a friend, photographer Richard Augustus, and a local pro-life doctor to oversee the photographing of the grisly scene."[1]

Right to Life of Kansas released those unforgettable photos in a brochure entitled "Our Throw Away Society." Later, according to the brochure, it was revealed that the hospital, under a contract from the city of Wichita, had for several years been sending the bodies of aborted and stillborn infants to that incinerator, which was owned by the city. There the babies' bodies were burned along with dogs, cats, and other animal remains from the pound next door. According to the brochure, when the mayor of Wichita was confronted with the evidence he said, "I know there needs to be a more dignified way to dispose of fetal tissues."[2]

"Fetal tissue?" All right, Mr. Mayor, lets look at that issue one more time. That is not "fetal tissue" you are incinerating. The word *fetus* in Latin simply means "young one" or "offspring." A fetus is a child, a son or daughter, a baby. But we have misused the Latin term these many years to hide us from reality. We want to think of a fetus in impersonal, technical terms. Review the evidence one more time. Decide for yourself if abortion is just removing and disposing of unwanted tissue or if, in fact, it is the murder of a baby.

We all learned in childhood that a male sperm unites at conception with a female ovum or egg. As a result of that fertilization process, the two cells become a single living cell, the size of a pinprick, smaller than a grain of sand,

63

smaller even than the period typed at the end of this sentence. During those first hours, twenty-three pairs of chromosomes from the mother and twenty-three pairs of chromosomes from the father come together carrying fifteen thousand genes from each parent cell. Those genes, in the words of Gary Bergel, executive director of Intercessors of America, "are like letters of a divine alphabet. They spell out the unique characteristics of the new individual. The color of the eyes, hair and skin, facial features, body type and qualities of personality and intelligence are all determined by this genetic coding."[3]

Read Gary Bergel's informative and inspired little pamphlet, *When You Were Formed in Secret,* or just pick up an encyclopedia or a book describing in clear, simple terms the process of birth. Most of us spend a lifetime not really knowing or understanding what goes on inside a mother's womb during those nine months of mystery. It is easy to kill what we do not know. Jennifer once said to me, "I didn't think of it as a baby; so it was easier to have my baby killed."

Jennifer and young women who are considering abortion need to understand the human being that is developing inside them. For a short time after the moment of conception Jennifer's baby didn't resemble anything human. As the fertilized egg divided into two cells, then into four cells and eight cells, the baby looked more like a raspberry. But that tiny cluster of growing cells already carried all the elements of the baby's final form as it traveled down the mother's Fallopian tube, entered the womb, and burrowed deep into the soft wall of her uterus. Growing and changing every hour, with each cell assigned a specific task, the child was mobilizing for a flurry of growth and development that staggers the imagination.

All of this happened without Jennifer even knowing a child was forming inside her.

Before Jennifer ever wondered if she were pregnant, the baby had formed a sack of water to live in, a life-support system called the amniotic fluid, which protects and supplies some nourishment to Jennifer's baby. The umbilical cord delivers food and disposes of waste materials. Inside that private universe, the embryo, a primitive but human form, was growing, changing, struggling to survive. By the time Jennifer had her pregnancy confirmed and decided to abort—if this had all happened within the first three or four weeks after conception—the embryo had formed a backbone, a spinal column, and a complete and complex nervous system. Simple kidneys, a liver, and a digestive system were taking shape within the child. The heart was already pulsating and pumping blood. Small buds, which would soon become arms and legs, were present. Eyes and ears had begun to form.

Only five weeks after conception, Jennifer's baby's brain began to develop. The head of the child was straightening up from its bent position and tiny hands and fingers had already appeared. During the sixth week, even the toes were visible. The baby's liver had taken over the production of his or her own blood cells. Brain waves could be detected, recorded, and even read by scientific instruments. The new child had his or her own circulatory, digestive, and waste eliminating systems. Eyelids had formed to cover much of the eyeballs. Soon, those eyelids closed and sealed shut to protect the developing light sensitive cells in the baby's eyes. Those eyelids would not open again until the seventh month of development.

During week seven, the child's complete skeleton began

to change from cartilage to true bone. Jaws formed, complete with teeth buds in the baby's gums. By the end of only eight weeks of growth, the baby had arms, elbows, forearms, and hands. Although the child was only one and one-eighth inches long and weighed approximately one thirtieth of an ounce, everything normal to human life had been established. The heart had been beating for a month and the body already responded to touch. Feeble movements could be recorded.

All this happened before Jennifer had missed two periods.

By the third month, Jennifer's pregnancy would begin to "show." The baby within her would double in length. Arms, hands, fingers, legs, feet, and toes would fully form. Even fingernails would begin to grow and fingerprints would appear. The heartbeat would be heard with a fetoscope. Genitals would show that the baby was a girl and would already contain primitive egg cells of their own. The baby would turn her head, curl and fan her toes, and open and close her mouth. She would sleep and awaken and "breathe" amniotic fluid regularly to exercise and develop her respiratory system. She would drink, digest, and excrete portions of the fluid.

Already she would know what she liked. When her amniotic fluid was sweetened, the baby would drink more. But when it was made bitter, the baby would drink less.

This is the person that the Supreme Court declared is not a person and thus has no legal right to life. Abortion is legal and accepted by many people during this first trimester.

During the fourth month, fine hair would begin to grow on the baby's head. Eyebrows and eyelashes would appear. The baby could suck her thumb. She would be six or seven inches long and already weigh approximately four ounces.

Her skin would be bright pink and transparent and covered with fine, downlike hair. Jennifer would feel her baby move. The baby's heart would pump up to twenty-five quarts of blood a day through her tiny system. Her life supporting umbilical cord, connected firmly to her mother's uterus, would carry three hundred quarts of fluid a day on a complete round trip from mother to baby to mother again in less than thirty seconds at speeds of up to four miles an hour.

In the fifth and sixth months, the baby would be ten to twelve inches long and weigh approximately one pound. Already, she could hear her mother's voice, rumblings in her mother's stomach, and the noises she made while eating or drinking. The baby could even hear outside noises. She could grasp her umbilical cord firmly. She could open and close her tiny fists. She could move gently at her own commands within her liquid nursery, waiting for the day she would make her decision to leave that secret sanctuary and make her way into the next stage of life outside the womb.

The Supreme Court has ruled that this baby, too, can be aborted.

Of course Jennifer's baby didn't reach the fifth month of development. She was aborted and her remains were disposed of by medical personnel during the sixth week. There would be no burial site where Jennifer could sit and meditate about her child's premature death. There would be no small monument for the courageous struggle for life the baby mounted until she died. The child would never have a name or a birthday to remember. There would be no pictures taken, no scrapbooks made to commemorate that short life.

How convenient it is. For if we remembered the aborted

babies, we would have to think about the way they died and the part that we as a nation played in killing them.

What I am about to describe to you next is as difficult for me to think about as it will be for you. Set in counterpoint against God's miracle of a child's creation and growth before birth is the destruction of that same innocent and helpless baby through the techniques of abortion. Before *Roe* v. *Wade*, I had never looked closely at the tools and the techniques of the abortionist. They were primarily illegal then anyway. Now that they're legal, we must see them for what they are.

Jennifer's doctor would select one of the five primary techniques used to abort a baby in the United States. However distasteful we find the discussion, we must remember that more than a half million teenagers like Jennifer chose to abort their babies last year in this country alone. It is as important to teach a teenager the truth about abortion as it is to explain the way a baby is conceived or develops within the mother's womb. Most women go in for an abortion with absolutely no information, let alone understanding the operation or its consequences for them or for their baby. Understanding how an abortion works may be the first step in preventing the abortion altogether.

Dilation and curettage has until recently been the method most often used to abort a baby during the first thirteen weeks of pregnancy. In this D & C surgery, the doctor inserts a tiny, hoelike instrument, the curette, into the womb through the dilated cervix. The abortionist scrapes the walls of the uterus, cutting the baby's body into removable pieces and extracting each piece as it is severed.

Picture it. The cervix, which is the neck or opening of the uterus, is closed tightly at the beginning of a pregnancy to seal the unborn baby safely in his or her sanctuary. The abortionist forces the cervix open prematurely, places the sharp tool into the uterus, breaks open the amniotic sac in which the baby is floating, and begins to hack away blindly at the unborn child growing there. As I will show you later in this chapter, well-supported scientific studies have proven that the baby feels pain from the sixth week of pregnancy; yet, the abortionist administers no anesthetic to kill or lessen the baby's pain. After a piece is torn or sliced from the child's body it is extracted through the cervix. Then the process begins again. There is a great deal of bleeding as the child dies. The head, usually too large to be removed through the cervix, must be crushed, and then the abortionist, still working blindly, gropes for the disembodied head with a long pair of surgical tweezers, pinching the ends together, and crushing whatever it finds until the baby's parts are removed and the abortion has finally ended.

Suction abortion has replaced dilation and curettage in many places and has become the most commonly used method for abortion of early pregnancies. This technique has simply added a powerful, vacuumlike device to the curette. The suction tube which resembles a straw is inserted through the cervix into the womb and the body of the unborn child and his placenta life support systems are torn to pieces and sucked into a container.

Dr. Bernard Nathanson, an obstetrician/gynecologist who once helped to found the National Abortion Rights Action League (NARAL), has filmed an actual suction abortion on a twelve-week child through ultrasound moving pictures to show the abortion from the child's perspective. The sonograms in this film, *The Silent Scream,* give graphic testimony to the tragic effectiveness of the suction device as it enters through the cervix and begins to cut and tear the baby's body into pieces small enough to be swallowed up by the suction device. This method, developed in the Republic of China, speeds up and somewhat simplifies the abortionist's task but doesn't allow any less pain or horror for its victim. In a late first trimester abortion the baby's head must still be found by blind probing and crushed by a surgical tool before it can be suctioned from the mother's womb.

After viewing Dr. Nathanson's film, the young doctor who had performed the abortion, an experienced abortionist with over ten thousand abortions to his credit, stopped performing abortions entirely. The young woman who operated the camera was an active feminist who spoke often on behalf of the pro-choice cause. After seeing the finished film, she quit speaking publicly on the subject of abortion altogether.

For me, the most devastating part of watching that suction abortion was not the silent scream seen sonographically on the tiny victim's face, but those first few seconds as the abortion begins. The suction device moves slowly through the cervix into the baby's quiet space. Suddenly, the child senses a mortal enemy and struggles to turn away. In that graphic moment there is no question that the baby is a human being who wants to survive and who is already given survival instincts. But against that deadly abortion tool, there is no escape. As we watch, the baby dies. His body is torn into bloody fragments. His head is crushed and the fragments are suctioned away.

Saline poisoning or *hypernatremic* abortions are generally used after thirteen weeks of pregnancy. A powerful salt solution is injected into the amniotic fluid in which the baby is floating. The needle bearing the saline solution is inserted through the mother's abdomen into the water sac. As the baby breathes and swallows the toxic liquid, she dies. Her death is slow and painful. She is strangled and her skin is blackened by the poison. Approximately twenty-four hours later, the mother goes into labor and discharges a burned, shriveled, grotesque corpse.

I have seen too many pictures of the children who were killed by this method. At night, when I close my eyes, I can picture them sleeping in the safety of that wonderful floating world only to be awakened by the sudden horror of their environment's being poisoned with no way to escape it. I picture them writhing in pain for hours. Even the gas chambers of Dachau were more humane and effective in administering death suddenly and by surprise. But there is another horror I connect with this salt poisoning technique. I have also seen pictures of the babies who have survived it and were born alive, still strangling on the poison, skin burned black and shriveled.

Hysterotomy or *caesarean section* abortions are used in the last three months of pregnancy. The womb is entered by surgery through the wall of the abdomen. The unborn baby is removed and allowed to die by neglect or by an overt act of murder.

Again horror stories abound. Doctors who have removed living children in an abortion are seldom taken to trial, much less found guilty and punished when their neglect or their overt actions cause a baby's death. Pro-life groups across America have been collecting stories of living babies found in hospital and clinic trash collectors, of babies left on tables and countertops to die, of babies strangled after a live birth. There are other well-documented cases of living babies being removed from their mothers during an abortion and sold to pathologists and scientists for experimentation.[4]

"Some 500 children every year survive the abortion process," reports the Center for Disease Control.[5] "And those children can be dealt with as chattel (property to be bought and sold)", adds Representative Christopher Smith (R-NJ).[6]

One notorious case that proves the congressman's fears is the research work of Dr. Peter A. Adams of Case Western Reserve University. Twelve second-trimester children aborted alive by hysterotomy were connected to a fluid circulating apparatus for experimentation.[7] Although there has been more and more legislation introduced to limit the problem of experimenting with the children who survive the abortion and are born alive, the problem continues.

Prostaglandin chemical abortion is the newest legal abortion technique available. A hormone is injected into the uterus causing it to contract intensely. The unborn child, waiting to be born at the appropriate time, is suddenly wrenched from his temporary life support system and pushed by the uterus from his sanctuary inside his mother's womb.

This new chemical, developed by the Upjohn Pharmaceutical Company, has its own history of abuse. Babies have survived the abortion attempt and have been born prematurely unequipped to face life, struggling to survive, hurt and handicapped by the abortion process. Babies not so fortunate have been decapitated by the sudden, violent birth. Mothers, too, have suffered from side effects caused by the new chemical and a number have even died from cardiac arrest following its use.[8]

The Upjohn Company lists the most ironic "complication" of all on the label of this chemical: "A live baby" is a possible complication.

There are many millions of women who will take the risks to themselves in order to abort an unwanted pregnancy, but when they hear that the abortion may cause their baby great pain, they hesitate. Most girls or women considering an abortion have no idea that their unborn baby will feel pain. Many doctors who perform abortions still do not believe it. Do you believe that the unborn child feels pain during the abortion procedure? Would it make a difference if you did?

On January 30, 1984, President Reagan, speaking before the National Religious Broadcasters convention that I was attending, said, "Medical science doctors confirm that when the lives of the unborn are snuffed out, they often feel pain, pain that is long and agonizing."

Again, on March 6, 1984, the president said, "...when abortions are being performed, the unborn children being killed often feel excruciating pain."[9] President Reagan does not claim to be an expert in fetology but he was quoting documented research.

The day after the president's first speech, Dr. Ervin Nichols, director of Practice Activities for the American College of Obstetricians and Gynecologists, an organization that has traditionally supported the practice of abortion, denied the president's claim that the child being killed by the abortionist feels pain. "We are unaware of any evidence of any kind that would substantiate a claim that pain is perceived by a fetus," he said to the *New York Times*.[10]

On February 13, 1984, the president received a letter fully backing his claims on fetal pain by twenty-four prominent medical obstetricians and gynecologists. "Mr. President," the letter began, "in drawing attention to the capability of the human fetus to feel pain, you stand on firmly established ground."[11]

Eventually, the same Dr. Nichols who had attempted to deny the president's claims reconsidered his response and claimed he had been quoted out of context by the press. He told a *Washington Times* correspondent that he was talking of the development of the unborn during its first three months and probably the next month and a half. He said he was not a fetal surgeon and lacked both expertise and intimate knowledge of this field.[12]

Dr. Vincent Collins, professor of anesthesiology at Northwestern University and author of *Principles of Anesthesiology*, a standard text on the science of preventing pain, declares that as early as eight weeks, and certainly by thirteen weeks of gestation, unborn human beings are pain sensitive.[13]

Finally, what about the effect of abortion upon the women who have this procedure? Few pregnant women realize the physical and emotional hazards of abortion.

Abortion is dangerous. There have been hundreds of controlled studies throughout the world on the effects of abortion on the women whose babies are aborted. After reviewing the physical and psychological damage that abortions can cause, many nations have made them illegal or have severely limited their accessibility.

I am especially indebted to John Lippis, author of the booklet, *The Challenge to Be 'Pro-Life,'* for reviewing the large collection of literature on this subject and organizing it for easy reading and understanding.[14]

Most American hospitals or abortion clinics perform so many abortions that follow-up and careful analysis of the results are difficult if not impossible to determine. Therefore, because there may be no obvious immediate or short-term complications, doctors and health officials who perform and administer abortions and the women who become casualties of abortion assume that abortions are safe. In fact, the long-term complications of abortions on their unsuspecting victims can be enormous.

Those long-term complications are especially dangerous to three kinds of women: young women, women in their first pregnancy, and women who wish to bear a child later. Jennifer fulfills all three categories. So do most of the estimated half-million teenagers who used abortion as a birth control method during 1984. So what are the dangers of abortion to Jennifer and to the teenagers, to the young women facing their first pregnancy, and to the women who want a baby some day, but not the baby they are carrying?

Abortion is dangerous to the body of a woman. Immediate physical complications may result from an abortion even if those who sell the process deny them or underplay them significantly. The statistics that I will use to support the reality of these complications are from the "Wynn Report," an analysis of seventy-five studies done in nations around the world by scientists who were neutral about the moral or medical consequences of the abortion procedures.[15]

Hemorrhaging (the discharge of blood as from a ruptured blood vessel) is predictable in 1 to 17 percent of the women who have a D & C or suction abortion during the first three months (twelve weeks) of pregnancy. According to Dr. Thomas Hilger's study entitled "Induced Abortion," heavy bleeding requiring a blood transfusion happens "usually" in 2 to 5 percent of all such abortions.[16]

Laceration of the cervix was reported in 4 to 5 percent of similar D & C or suction abortions. According to the *British Medical Journal*, the rough, jagged tearing process caused by the forced entry of the surgical instrument into the womb causes nearly half of the women lacerated to lose their next wanted baby through miscarriage if the attending physican does not reinforce the cervix with a special suture during the next pregnancy.[17]

Perforation of the uterus itself is reported in only .5 to 1 percent of the cases studied.[18] Cutting accidentally through the delicate wall of the uterus can cause peritonitis, the inflammation of the membrane lining of the abdominal cavity.

Infections, from mild to serious occur in 2 to 19 percent of the women who aborted, depending on the study you read.[19]

Cases of hepatitis from blood transfusions received during an abortion are growing more common. As our blood supply problem increases with the growing epidemic of AIDS (Acquired Immune Deficiency Syndrome), every blood transfusion for any reason creates a real risk.

Blood clots and emboli (tiny undissolved particles of matter) may get into the bloodstream and be carried and deposited by it to various parts of the body resulting in a variety of ill effects ranging from minimal to quite serious.

Anesthetic death is a hazard listed without percentages. But anyone undertaking a surgical procedure involving anesthesia takes a risk. Abortions requiring anesthesia are no exception.

John Lippis reminds us that "an abortionist operates completely blind in this surgery, working by touch alone. If he manipulates the curette...too easily or too forcibly, harm will be done to the woman."[20] A study from the prestigious British medical journal *Lancet* by the abortionists themselves shows that in 1,182 of their suction abortion procedures, they found that 9.5 percent of their patients required blood transfusion, 4.2 percent suffered cervical lacerations, 1.2 percent had uterine perforations, and 27 percent developed infections.[21] These complications are seldom mentioned by those who claim abortion is safe.[22]

Long-term physical complications from the abortion process are harder to measure but no less significant. Miscarriage may result to half the women whose cervix is lacerated during the surgery. Damage to the Fallopian tubes or the lining of the womb and the general weakening of the cervix may lead to sterility. According to international studies, the range of possibility for sterility resulting from an abortion is between 2 and 5 percent, although studies in Czechoslovakia are as high as 25 percent; Finland—15 percent; Japan—10 percent; and Poland—7 percent. According to a recent study of over 5,000 delivered babies, those women with prior induced abortions had a 7 to 15 percent increased prevalence of placenta previa during the next delivery, a serious complication which may lead to serious bleeding during labor and may require a Caesarean section to save the baby's life.

There is increasing proof that abortions greatly affect the miscarriage and premature birth rate in the wanted pregnancies that follow. Mr. Lippis demonstrates that "there is double to triple the normal incidence of first trimester miscarriages after a previous abortion."[23] Other studies show, Lippis says, "that the rate of miscarriages in the second trimester (12–24 weeks of pregnancy) are two, six and even ten times that of pregnancies without prior abortions." Lippis adds, "The possibilities of premature birth (the primary cause of infant death in the first month, and one of the leading causes of mental and motor retardation) are increased 40 percent after one abortion and 70 percent after two."[24]

I am using Lippis's extensive survey of the physical effects of abortion on women because there is too much data for a lay scientist like myself to read, digest, and report back. I also believe that the pro-life forces are more trustworthy in the reading and interpreting of the data because they have only one goal, the saving of the children. I find it as difficult to trust the advocates of abortion with their defense of abortion as I did to trust the tobacco companies with their findings that disputed the surgeon general's report that smoking may cause cancer.

As I study the statistics pouring in from across the nation and around the world, I am increasingly convinced of the terrible variety of immediate and long-term dangers of abortion. The abortion industry has much to lose if this information gets to the general public. Already, this data is under massive attack by the doctors and clinics and pro-choice agencies who support abortion. The least the Supreme Court could do after making its tragic blunder is to cause every doctor, hospital, clinic, public health agency, school counselor, parent, teacher, or friend who advocates abortion to post a caution not unlike the caution posted on every cigarette pack or advertisement.

WARNING
ABORTIONS MAY KILL BABIES, THEIR MOTHERS,
AND THEIR BROTHERS AND SISTERS YET UNBORN.

Abortions are dangerous to the mind and spirit of a woman. As Jennifer continues to share her own deeply moving story, it will become more and more obvious how devastating abortion can be on the emotional as well as the physical state of the woman who decides to abort her baby. There are millions of stories like Jennifer's and there will be at least four thousand more in this country during the next twenty-four hours. That could mean another 1.5 million abortions during the next twelve months. It is time we spoke frankly of these stories of the women who will begin an almost certain time of emotional suffering after their unborn children are aborted.

Almost every woman we have interviewed through Liberty Godparent Ministries reports a long and painful struggle with guilt for having made the decision to abort her baby in the first place. And, though painful, it was easier to deal with that guilt as long as it was generally held that what had been aborted was just a "lifeless," "shapeless," "unfeeling" piece of tissue. Now the evidence is in. An abortion kills a living baby with arms and legs, fingers and toes, heart and brain and body.

Women who chose abortion speak of seeing the faces of their babies in living children on the street or in the playgrounds. They hear their babies calling out to them. They dream of holding their aborted babies in their arms, and they awaken feeling all the grief and loss that any death in a family brings to those who remain. They report nightmares that dramatize the moments of their babies' deaths and the horrors of knowing the parts they played in the sufferings. Others spend months, years, even a lifetime denying the baby even existed. This kind of tragic, debilitating guilt may lead a woman to all kinds of neurotic, even psychotic disorders.

The loneliness that may follow the loss of the unborn

child is often compounded by the loss of a relationship with the man or boy who fathered the child. I have read that 70 percent of the relationships that produced the aborted baby fail within one month after the abortion. That may sound like good news to a parent who has gone through an abortion experience with a daughter, but the results of the loneliness that follows this double loss may lead to a pendulum swing of emotions that begins the entire abortion process once again.[25]

A study in the *British Medical Journal* shows that 43 percent of women who aborted were pregnant again within the year following their abortion.[26] Jennifer's story is typical of those suffering from guilt. The act of having another child may be a conscious or unconscious attempt to undo what has been done through the abortion. It is also typical of those suffering from loneliness who attempt to find another man or boy get pregnant again by him as a conscious or unconscious attempt to end the loneliness and recapture intimacy lost because of the abortion.

Women who are sensitive, who may have had emotional crises or disorders previous to their abortions, are especially vulnerable to the emotional anguish that often follows. Ironically, most girls and women decide to have an abortion because of the "mental anguish" being created by the unwanted pregnancy. Yet, few get frank, helpful counseling as to the mental anguish they will experience following the abortion and in varying degrees for the rest of their lives.

Most of the women who are emotionally damaged by an abortion are numbered among the walking wounded. They lead active lives. The suffering in their minds and spirits is manageable. Many find the remedy for their guilt in God's love and forgiveness and the remedy for loneliness in God's people and their concern. But there are other abortion victims whose emotional anguish never heals. The guilt and loneliness drive them to despair. They seek forgiveness from others but never seem able to forgive themselves. Their despair becomes self-destructive. Often alcohol and drug misuse lead to further suffering.

Studies show that in some cases postabortion emotional trauma may lead to serious emotional breakdowns and even to suicide.

In the November 1981 issue of *Pediatrics*, Carl L. Tishler, Ph. D., alerts doctors "to the possibility that a teenager who has had an induced abortion, may attempt to kill herself on the day which corresponds to her baby's birthday had the baby been allowed to be born."[27] After a thorough study of the data, John Lippis warns that "abortion is linked to recent increases in female and teenage suicide."[28] He quotes Dr. Ben Sheppard, physician and juvenile court judge, who wrote in the *British Medical Journal*, "Young adolescents who have had abortions may verbalize relief, but their internal feeling is psychic trauma and loss of personal morality which will persist throughout life."[29]

Making the choice between killing the baby or living through the pregnancy and giving the baby birth may be the most difficult decision a woman ever has to make. No one should ever minimize the terror and the loneliness of that awful, life-changing decision. But I am convinced that the physical and emotional risks to the woman who decides to kill the baby are far worse than the physical and emotional risks the woman takes to let the baby live.

The woman who decides upon abortion may be harmed physically and emotionally. The unborn baby is killed. Who benefits from abortion?

5

A Recurring Nightmare

JENNIFER

"Where are you going?" my father asked, looking up from his newspaper as I carried two suitcases and a hanging bag toward the door.

"Over to Shelly's, Dad," I answered, leaning over to kiss him on the cheek. "I'll be staying there while you are in Washington, and Mom is in Florida."

"Will you be careful, Jennifer?" Mom added as she came in from the bedroom where she had been packing for her long-awaited vacation.

"Careful enough," I answered rather sharply without even looking in her direction.

Something awful had begun to happen between my mother and me during those last two years in high school. I knew she loved me and I loved her, but every conversation between us quickly became a shouting match. I didn't understand her. She didn't understand me. Somewhere along the way we both gave up trying to understand each other. We just yelled across the distance between us and the distance grew wider and wider as we yelled. Slowly, almost without noticing, my best friend had become my enemy.

"Careful enough isn't an answer," she said loudly. "I want a promise that while we're gone you'll…"

"Mom," I shouted, turning to face her. "I'm not a child anymore. I'm a high school graduate. I'm eighteen years old."

I reached for the door, hoping my little outburst would silence her. It only made her angry. She walked quickly to the door and placed her hand on it to block my exit.

"Jennifer," she said, taking a deep breath and trying to stay calm. "You may have your own life, but as long as you live it under our roof you will obey our rules. We don't like your going out every night."

"I haven't been going out every night," I interrupted her.

"Let me finish," she said with exaggerated calm. "We don't know where you go or what you do out there, but we do know that almost every night you come home smelling of beer and stale cigarettes."

"That's not true," I yelled back, looking to my father for support. "I don't come in all that late, Dad." I ignored my mother altogether. "And I don't smell!"

Dad just looked at the two of us sadly. He had watched our relationship deteriorate over the past few months. He knew that mother-daughter warfare was common during the late teen years, but he knew, too, that our warfare was getting out of hand and he didn't know what to do about it. He loved us both and felt sad and helpless as he watched us grow more and more hostile toward each other.

Looking back now it is easier to see what had been happening between us. During my junior and senior years, in spite of the good times and successes, I had become more and more unhappy. I was easily irritated and often depressed. I felt lonely most of the time. Shelly was good company, but I needed more than girl talk and giggles. Something had gone wrong in my life. I didn't know then what it was, but I knew that I was miserable and angry and lonely most of the time. And I desperately needed someone or something to make me feel good again.

So I dated and went to parties. I did what all the kids were doing our junior and senior years. I had been awkward and skinny and embarrassed long enough. It felt good to have guys interested in me. I loved to be out with them so I didn't have to face the tension at home. It was a vicious circle. The less I was home, the more trouble I got into and the more trouble I got into, the less I wanted to be at home. Instead of being with my family I spent a lot of nights with friends where there was no one to tell me what to do and what not to do.

"Jennifer," my mother said quietly that day, reaching out to touch me as she spoke. "You have been drinking at these parties and the last few nights you've been drinking too much. Think where that could lead," she said.

I jerked my arm back from my mother's hand, walked quickly to the door, and turned to face her. Her face was flushed. Her eyes were blinking back the tears. Her hands were clenched. She was right. We both knew it. I had been drinking at those parties. I liked the way I felt after a couple of drinks. A beer or two helped me kill those awful feelings I wanted to avoid. I laughed more. I loosened up. I felt free.

"I'll drink if I want to drink," I whispered fiercely.

"Yes, and you'll use drugs, too, I suppose," Mother shouted back.

"Drugs?" I yelled. "You think I'm using drugs?"

"One thing leads to another, Jennifer," she answered. "And God knows where it will all end."

I stared at her for one long, angry moment. Then, without answering, I pushed open the door and stormed out into the driveway. Our fights always seemed to end with my mother's not-so-subtle implications. "Where will it lead?" I knew what she had in mind. We all did. We never spoke of the abortion, but it was always there hanging over us like a black storm cloud. We tried to ignore it but it wouldn't go away. We tried to forget it but it crowded our memories and haunted our dreams. I didn't realize it then, but the abortion was a turning point for all of us. I think now that my four hours in that abortion clinic was the beginning of a long list of troubles for our family, including my growing depression and my parents' growing fears.

I walked quickly down the driveway, slid behind the wheel of my Volkswagen beetle, and turned the key.

"Start, you little creep," I muttered as the engine turned over once and died. I wanted to get away before our fight began again. Sometimes my mother and her warnings followed me out the door, down the sidewalk, and up to the car without pausing. I could see her standing in the doorway looking at me as I turned the key again. All I could think of was getting away from her angry voice.

I wish now that I could have known where my rebellion was leading me. It had all begun innocently enough. I had been lonely and depressed in high school after Mike graduated. We had become close friends. We dated regularly. He loved me and I loved him. When he graduated and went away to college, there was a short time when we managed to keep our relationship alive. Then the letters quit coming and the visits stopped. We never ended our friendship formally. But I knew by his silence that it was over.

My senior year was a difficult, lonely time. I needed

someone to love me. My mom and dad loved me, but their love wasn't enough. Shelly loved me, but we were just girlhood chums. Then I met Jeff and I thought maybe this time someone would love me enough to make the hurting go away.

I don't know why Jeff and I kept noticing each other at parties, except that I was without Mike and Jeff was almost always alone. He had the most beautiful eyes of anyone I had ever seen. They were so dark, and so deep-set that they looked black, and they sparkled when he talked. He used to wear black jeans with blue-and-white checked Vans, a white T-shirt with the sleeves cut off, and an old leather flight jacket that had belonged to his dad who died in Vietnam. He looked like James Dean in one of those black-and-white posters from *Giant*. He was quiet and often sat staring into the fire for hours at a time. Then his mood would change and we would go racing across the back roads in his dad's old jeep. I loved the way Jeff held me when we danced or lay on the floor watching videos in Shelly's basement game room.

I grinned to myself even as I struggled to start the flooded motor. Dad was going to an important conference in Washington. Mom was taking time to visit her sister in Florida for the first time in years. They would be gone for three weeks. I needed to stay in town to keep my summer job. Three whole weeks without my mother's warning threats. Three whole weeks in Shelly's great house. Three whole weeks with Jeff.

I liked the way I felt when I was with him. When he kissed me or held my face in his hands and said, "I love you," I felt the loneliness and the depression fade away. He loved me. I loved him. Though I really believed that making love should be saved for marriage, I broke my rules with Jeff. I swore the first time would be the last. The second time was easier. Time sped by. The Senior Prom, final exams, graduation, and summer vacation were a whirlwind and Jeff was the quiet center of the storm. Jeff and I had big plans for those next three parent-free weeks.

Shelly was waiting for me outside her parents' sprawling home in a suburb near the mountains. She jumped down from her perch on the ranch-style fence that encircled their property and raced toward my little Volkswagen bug.

"Jennifer!" she yelled.

I parked the car and ran toward her, giggling.

"Three weeks," I said. "I can't believe it."

Shelly's parents were good people, but they both had careers. Shelly's dad was an architect, her mom an interior decorator. They were often gone on projects together until late at night or even for days at a time. For the next three weeks we would have the run of the house and could entertain our friends there in total privacy. Mom called from Florida the next night to see if everything was all right. I had been having strange little cramps in my abdomen, but they didn't seem worth mentioning to Shelly, much less to Mother. I was so happy to be on my own at last and I certainly didn't want to mess things up right from the start.

Every day the cramps got worse. During the first week at Shelly's I was awakened by sharp pains in my stomach and abdomen. When I felt my abdomen, I noticed swelling. I suspected cancer. It was common in our family.

One morning the pains doubled me over onto the cold tile floor in the bathroom Shelly and I were sharing. I have never been a trooper, my mother says, when it comes to pain. Shelly found me kneeling there, clutching my stomach and groaning in pain.

We had a party scheduled for that night. Jeff was coming. I could not be sick.

At that very moment the telephone rang. It was Dad, calling from Washington just to see how we were doing.

"Tell him, Jennifer," Shelly whispered as I picked up the phone. "Or I'll tell him myself."

She started for the extension phone in her room. I cupped my hand over the telephone mouthpiece and whispered loudly, "Get away from that phone, traitor. I'll tell him."

Toward the middle of our conversation, I mentioned the abdominal pains. At first I made light of them, but when Dad questioned me further, I admitted that the symptoms made me wonder about cancer.

My father said to hang up and he would call a doctor who was a friend of his. Only five minutes later, he called me back to say, "You have an appointment at ten o'clock this morning."

Shelly drove us into town. She sat in the waiting room and stared at an old *National Geographic* while I went in for the emergency checkup. There was something growing in me, all right. The ultrasound test proved that, but it wasn't cancer.

"It's a baby," I told Shelly, as we staggered arm-in-arm out of the waiting room into the noontime sun.

"A baby?" Shelly echoed wearily. "You're pregnant? Again?"

We barely made it to the car before I burst into tears. Shelly drove quickly toward her home trying to comfort me as we moved through those familiar city streets. Everything I saw made me cry harder—the high school, my church, Jeff's street.

This time I had taken birth control pills as the doctor had suggested after the abortion. But every once in a while I had forgotten. *How could I?* I wondered.

Shelly helped me into the living room and I lay back on a huge stuffed chair and sobbed until the tears were gone. She brought me a piece of tissue and a glass of water and waited for me to calm down.

"I know what we'll do," she said when I finally got control again. "We'll get an apartment together somewhere out of state. I'll get a job and you can have the baby."

I listened while my friend concocted a crazy plan. She was serious. She wanted me to keep the baby this time, and she wanted to help me keep it. But I would not allow my best friend to leave her home and family to get a job somewhere as a waitress to support my baby while I lived on welfare. I was too practical to accept her offer and too angry.

The first time I got pregnant, I was innocent. I didn't understand anything. I was just hurt and frightened. But the second time I got pregnant, I also got angry. I was angry at the first man who made me pregnant without loving me. I was angry at Jeff who said he loved me but made me pregnant anyway.

"Why did he do it?" I muttered through my tears. "Why wasn't he more careful?"

Shelly listened silently as I just babbled accusations at Jeff. "He'll get off scot-free," I remember shouting at Shelly that day. "I'll have to pay the price."

I didn't call Jeff. I didn't tell him that I was pregnant. In fact, he still doesn't know. I don't remember exactly why I left him out of my decision. I was angry, afraid, and deceitful all at once. I knew I didn't want to marry him. I knew that would be wrong. So, I walked away and faced the problem without him.

Suddenly, I felt very much alone. Suddenly, those three weeks of freedom looked like a bad mistake. I was tired of freedom. I wanted my parents back. I knew I had to call my dad and tell him the doctor's diagnosis.

"Dad?" I could hear his voice over the long distance line. I knew how awful he felt as he waited to hear the results of the doctor's test. But I couldn't speak. I didn't have the courage to tell him.

"Jen," he finally said. "Are you pregnant?"

"I'm going to Florida," I answered, ignoring his question completely. "Tomorrow. To see Mom. I'll call you from there."

"Jen," he said again, "it's all right. Everything is all right. Don't worry."

Suddenly, I began to cry again, gripping the phone for dear life and sobbing long distance as Dad, a thousand miles away, waited for me to get control of myself.

"I saw a television special just yesterday," he finally said to me, "about a maternity home in Virginia where you can have your baby in privacy. They take care of everything, even an adoption. There was a number to call. I'll find it and call you back."

"A place in Virginia..." I moaned as Shelly hung up the phone and helped me lie back on a living room sofa. "...where I can save my baby? Great."

I pictured a haunted house with army nurses and big needles and pregnant girls behind locked doors and barred windows. I remembered Charles Dickens and David Copperfield and orphanages with huge gates and cobwebs. I saw myself alone and in labor in a place far from anyone who loved me.

"Give me that phone," I said to Shelly. "I'm going to call Mom. I'm going to Florida, tomorrow. She'll know what to do."

The drive to Florida was endless. It's a miracle I made it there alive. I cried from Macon, Georgia, on Interstate 75 South all the way to the Florida state line. I cried through Perry and Tifton and Valdosta. I cried until my eyes hurt and my throat was sore. I cried six hours until I reached my aunt's home in Baldwin, a little town outside Jacksonville where my mom and her sister were waiting.

I hadn't told her about my pregnancy on the telephone. I was too afraid. She had warned me so many times during those last two years of high school. Her words, "Where will it lead?" haunted me on that midnight ride to Jacksonville. But as I drove through the darkened streets of Baldwin looking for Aunt Elizabeth's home, I knew that Mom would be outside, waiting for me.

"I've been worried sick," she said walking down the drive to meet me. "What's wrong?"

She put her arm around me and led me toward the house. We sat on a screened-in back porch. For a moment I forgot the tension between us. We sat on a swing seat. She held me and rocked me back and forth gently waiting for me to speak, knowing what I would say. It was too late to begin the war between us once again. We postponed the loud, angry words during those next twenty-four hours and tried to solve my problem.

"I saw a television special," Mom said finally after I had poured out my calamity to her.

"About a place in Virginia?" I finished her sentence sarcastically.

"Yes," she said surprised, "how did you know?"

"Dad told me about it on the phone," I answered. "Oh, please, Mom," I blurted out, "don't make me go to one of those places."

For the next hour over iced tea and key lime pie my mother talked to me about a Reverend Jerry Falwell and his maternity home in Virginia. She had been devoted to "The Old-Time Gospel Hour" for several years. She had known about Liberty Godparent Ministries from the beginning. She had heard moving stories about girls like myself who had gone to Virginia to save their babies and she was sure it was the answer.

"There's no way you're going to get me to move into some weird home for unwed mothers," I said, thinking she had gone crazy on me. "There's just no way."

In spite of my protests and my angry replies, Mom didn't give in. She and Dad had talked about it already. They had decided. Now they were just waiting for me to be convinced. For two days she told me about Jerry Falwell and Lynchburg, Virginia, and the Liberty Godparent Home. She tried to convince me to go there and to find out for myself. I listened and remained unconvinced.

"Just think about it," she said growing more and more exasperated by my resistance. "Call them. Talk to them. Please."

Mom and I had reached an impasse, yet we couldn't talk about anything else. We had gone round and round until I could stand it no more. Even though it was almost eleven o'clock at night, I decided to leave for home. I would not listen to Mom's pleas to stay until morning.

I left Mom and Aunt Elizabeth at 11:00 in the evening the night after I arrived in Jacksonville.

I hugged Mom before I drove away. Not once had she

said, "I told you so." Not once had she scolded me.

I didn't want to go to that awful place I pictured in a God-forsaken little backwater town in the hills of the Appalachians. I didn't want to get mixed up with a television preacher and his spooky old maternity home. But my mother had at least suggested a solution.

"There must be another way," I said to her as I was leaving. "And if there is I'll find it."

Everyone had reacted so differently to my second pregnancy. The first time everyone had quickly decided an abortion was the only answer. But after going through it together and after living with what we had done for more than two years, our ideas had changed completely. No one really admitted it, but everyone felt the same. The guilt and grief from having one abortion was enough. No one mentioned it again. Still, I couldn't imagine having a baby. I wasn't married. I didn't have a job or an apartment. I planned on college and a career.

Sixty minutes after I left Jacksonville, in the middle of nowhere on a dark and empty highway, my faithful little Volkswagen beetle began to sputter and lose power in the fast lane where I'd been driving. I pulled quickly across the highway and coasted down the nearest off-ramp to the only twenty-four-hour station I noticed on the long and lonely drive.

It was past midnight and no mechanic was available until morning. I called Shelly and locked myself into the Volkswagen to await her arrival.

The night was endless. There was no moon. No stars. No midnight visions. I just sat in the scary silence watching a beautiful moth fly around and around a hot light that hung above the gas station. The moth was black and gold and fuzzy. Its wings were irridescent blue. As I watched I wondered why such a beautiful creature didn't have sense enough to fly away to safety. It fluttered and danced about the light closer and closer until with a terrible sizzling sound, it died and fell into a heap with all the others.

Lying on the back seat of a locked Volkswagen with the door handle jammed into my back and my feet curled under me, I pictured myself fluttering and dancing about the light. I determined that this time I would be smart enough to fly away to safety.

That awful night was one of the best things that ever happened to me. There beside that filling station in the middle of nowhere, something changed within me. I grew up.

"Dear, Lord," I prayed. "Please help me." I hadn't prayed for a long time, not a real prayer, not like this one. "I'm in bad trouble again, Lord, and I don't know what to do about it." I stared into the darkness trying to find God out there. "Help me know if I should go to this Godparent Home place, or help me find some better way."

I lay in the darkness praying and crying and thinking about that once-beautiful moth for the rest of the night. At 6:00 A.M. Shelly finally arrived. We drove home together in silence.

Exhausted when we finally turned into Shelly's driveway, we went right to bed, only to be awakened a short time later by the telephone. "Jen, this is Dad," the voice said from somewhere far away.

"Dad?" I asked coming wide awake.

"Mom and I are both catching planes within the next hour. We'll be home by noon. We've talked all night about your baby. We know you don't want to go to Lynchburg, but..."

"I'll go," I interrupted.

For a moment there was silence.

"You will?" he said, sounding surprised that I had offered no argument against their plan.

"Yes, Dad," I answered. "I want to go."

I was as surprised about my attitude change as he was. All my resistance had been drained away the night before.

"Go home then," he instructed me, "and get your clothes ready. I'm proud of you, Jen."

6

Is There a Better Way?

JERRY

"Is it enough to be against abortion?" the young reporter had asked me. "What are you doing for the pregnant girls who have no other options?"

I will never forget the press conference when that bright young newswoman confronted me with her question. From that moment I worked to find a way to help those other victims of abortion, the girls and women facing unwanted pregnancies. Fortunately, I had been open to her question. Unfortunately, my response didn't happen overnight. Although the direction of my life has been changed by my struggle to stop the killing of the nation's unborn babies and to give pregnant girls and women a chance to save their babies, the process has been long and painful.

In the years between this confrontation and the *Roe* v. *Wade* decision, I had traveled across the country. I had met pro-life leaders and volunteers from every strata of society. There were Catholics, Protestants, and Jews dedicated to saving the unborn, and there were agnostics and atheists equally committed to the cause. I met men and women who were white and black, yellow and brown, rich and poor, who had university degrees and who were self-taught, who were powerful and famous and who were without political clout. They all shared the same determination to save the children.

We had other issues in common besides the pro-life issue. We were committed to the traditional family. We were opposed to illegal drug traffic and the proliferation of pornography. We believed in free enterprise and a strong national defense. Color or class or creed made no difference when it came to the priorities that we shared. We were Americans who believed that our nation was in big trouble, and we were naive enough to think that we could do something about it.

One day in 1979 in a hotel room in Lynchburg, Virginia, I was meeting with a group of pro-life leaders from across the country. At the luncheon break, Paul Weyrich looked across the table at me and said, "Jerry, there is in America a moral majority that agrees about the basic issues. But they aren't organized. They don't have a platform. The media ignore them. Somebody's got to get that moral majority together."

Suddenly, a bell went off in my head. Paul was thinking lower case *m* when he said "moral majority," but it was the perfect name for a new organization that would bring together the people who believed in this nation, who were willing to work to preserve and protect her future.

What I didn't realize was that a nucleus of those people had already been gathered. Millions of those who agreed about these basic issues listened to me regularly on radio or watched me every Sunday on television's "Old Time Gospel Hour." We had their names and addresses in our computer. As I had traveled across the nation as a preacher and teacher, I had met tens of thousands of them in person.

In 1976, for example, a patriotic team of singers, actors, and musicians from our Liberty University campus trucked and bused to 141 cities across the nation. During the bicentennial year, seventy students in colorful patriotic costumes accompanied us on patriotic rallies in coliseums from New York to Los Angeles. Everywhere we appeared, the people mobbed us. They came to hear the young people's *America Back to God* musical presentation and my message calling America to repentance. They applauded their approval of our plea to return to those basic tenets upon which our nation was built. They joined in singing the great songs of this land and stood to their feet when the flag was raised and the national anthem sung. We had experienced the power and promise of this great silent majority and we had gathered their names and addresses in every city along the way.

When Paul Weyrich had described that moral majority, just waiting to be offered an opportunity to work on behalf of the issues that could save the nation, it triggered in me a feeling that had been growing since the Supreme Court's decision to legalize abortion on January 22, 1973. The nation needed an organization that could stand up to the power brokers, to the special interest lobbies, to the "good ole boy" politicians, and to the liberal media on behalf of the unborn children and the other causes we held in common.

By June 1979, with the help of lawyers in our nation's capital, we organized as the Moral Majority, Incorporated, a 501C4 political lobbying organization, and the Moral Majority Foundation, a 501C3 educational foundation. The purposes of the foundation were to publish a newspaper, produce and broadcast radio and television programs, conduct seminars, and generally support the work of the Moral

Majority as it mobilized members and volunteers in every village, town, city, county, and state in the nation.

Occasionally a Christian publication criticizes the Moral Majority for not espousing Christian faith. We never intended the Moral Majority to be a religious organization. We didn't organize to support a religious or sectarian cause. We welcome all Americans to work on behalf of our nation's renewal. There is no religious affiliation required. We are united on the basis of our citizenship in this country and our commitment to shared moral views and values. We have joined together representing every race, religion, and creed in the land for the express purpose of saving the country in this time of crisis. And though millions of born-again Christians like myself are members of the Moral Majority, it must not be confused with a religious organization. America has given each of us the freedom to believe or to not believe in religious tenets. The Moral Majority was founded to preserve and to protect that freedom.

My own personal pilgrimage from being a pastor against social activism before 1973 to becoming the founder of Moral Majority is in some ways similar to the history of my church on Thomas Road in Lynchburg, Virginia. Before 1973, we were like most Fundamentalist churches. We cared about the world in which we lived. We initiated projects to feed, clothe, and house the poor; collected seasonal offerings for special community services; and supported missionaries around the world. However, we saw ourselves as caring primarily about spiritual issues. We took a strong stand against abortion with clear, biblical teaching, but we didn't reach out to the pregnant girls in our community with a practical plan to help them save their babies until years after the Supreme Court's decision.

After *Roe* v. *Wade,* the people of Thomas Road Baptist Church, like their pastor, began to realize more and more that we were not doing enough to really help the suffering in our community. To talk about abortion was one thing. To help people actually facing the decision to abort was something else. Most of the girls and women we talked to didn't want to kill their babies, but they were ashamed and embarrassed by the predicament of their unwanted pregnancy. Often, they were rejected by parents and friends. Some wouldn't even have a place to live during their pregnancy or a way to support themselves if they chose to keep their baby. They were often young teenagers without a job, without a husband, without any means of support. They couldn't afford to pay for prenatal care, hospitalization, or the delivery of their baby. Others couldn't risk being fired from a job or being expelled from school. They didn't want to lose a boyfriend or feel his anger. They didn't know where to turn for help because practically everyone they knew—friends, family, teachers, counselors, boyfriends, employers—recommended abortion as the "quick and easy" way out of a very difficult problem. They ended up like Jennifer, victims of an abortion.

The people of Thomas Road Baptist Church spent years after *Roe* v. *Wade* trying to find the most effective way to help the girls and women in our community who were facing unwanted pregnancies. We offered counseling and some emergency services. We provided crisis aid to those who asked. We studied what other churches and communities were doing. We read and traveled, talked and prayed. It was not enough.

After waiting far too long, we finally established Phase One of our Liberty Godparent Ministries. Phase One included a crisis pregnancy center, "shepherding homes" (volunteer homes where mature women can live in privacy while awaiting their baby's birth), and an emergency hot line. The crisis pregnancy center of the Thomas Road Baptist Church offered free pregnancy tests to girls and women who wanted to confirm their suspicions about being pregnant without notifying family or friends. They needed a competent, non-judgmental place to be tested. By providing it, our staff and volunteers could be the first on the scene to help the person facing an unwanted pregnancy to decide about abortion. There was no question that our confidential pregnancy counseling had a goal in mind. We wanted to help stop the killing of unborn children. However, the center also counseled girls and women who had suffered through an abortion and were seeking guidance and forgiveness in a confidential atmosphere of Christian love and competence.

Volunteers from Thomas Road Baptist Church opened their homes to women awaiting the birth of their babies. Called "shepherding homes," these "homes away from home" provided a loving, Christian environment where a pregnant woman could find sanctuary during her months of unwanted pregnancy. While a woman awaited her child's birth, she could attend classes in child care and life skills taught by our staff and volunteers. This form of continuing education kept her mind and hands busy during the waiting season and helped prepare her for that day when she would be busy as a mother or back in the job force once again.

Perhaps the most dramatic dimension of this first phase of our program was our Godparent Centers. We organized and trained operators to receive calls from pregnant girls and women from around the country when they were faced with the same terrible choice that Jennifer had to make: to kill the baby or to let the baby live.

Working as a telephone operator on the crisis hot line is a sometimes frightening and always exhausting task. Operators know that the life of an unborn baby and the physical and mental health of a pregnant girl or woman may hang in the balance during that one call. Our experience with the hot line taught us that there is a brief forty-eight hour period in which the pregnant girl makes up her mind whether to abort or to save her baby. Usually when the girl calls, the abortion has been scheduled, the decision made. We have that one call to save the unborn child's life.

Last year our nationwide volunteers answered approximately one million crisis calls. Our hot line operators in Lynchburg alone answer an average of two thousand emergency calls a week. Now we employ paid operators as well as volunteers. Each is trained in handling emergencies skillfully. The phone banks are staffed in three shifts, twenty-four hours a day, seven days a week. Practically every call comes from a girl like Jennifer whose personal and confidential story could be the subject of a book. Each story is urgent, dramatic, and heart-rending. Many stories are stranger than fiction, unbelievable, even horrifying. In the following two stories, I've eliminated the girls' names for obvious reasons. This is a sample of the true stories of young women like Jennifer who call the Godparent Center's hot line every day. In some cases we succeed in our mission. In others the calls come too late.

From Baltimore, Maryland, a fourteen-year-old girl called the toll-free, crisis hot line. She was terrified. The operators could barely hear her whispered plea for help. In this first quick contact with the hot line, she confessed that her father was sexually abusing her on a regular basis and was using the girl and her two-year-old brother in pornographic films. She had waited to call until her father was too drunk to interrupt. She warned the operator not to call the police. Then, without giving her name or number, she suddenly hung up the phone.

All calls are held in strictest confidence unless our operator fears for the life or well-being of the woman calling. In this case our operators felt that the girl in Baltimore needed immediate aid. They notified the police and a child service office in Baltimore, putting them on standby in case the girl called again, and then notified members of Thomas Road Baptist Church to begin a prayer chain on behalf of the girl and her family.

Within the hour, the girl called again. The operator strained to hear the horror story as it unfolded further. "Last night my daddy killed my mommy," she whispered, "and he made me help him lift her body into the freezer."

This time the operator managed to get the girl's address. Police and social workers were notified and moved quickly to the scene, but the father shot and killed himself as they approached the house.

That tragic moment was the beginning of new life for the girl and for her little brother. They were placed with a Christian foster family through a city agency in Baltimore. The fourteen-year-old girl who had placed the call delivered a healthy baby, which was adopted by a Christian family. The girl then called a Godparent Center after her own child's adoption to thank the operators who had helped her when she needed it most.

The sixteen-year-old girl who called from Kansas City was another incest victim pregnant by her father. She had taken a handful of pills and was awaiting death. She called from a pay phone. The drugs were taking hold. She was gasping for breath. Her words were mumbled, her thoughts incoherent. The crisis was real.

Our Godparent Center hot line operators immediately notified Kansas City police while the girl was on the phone, but the dying girl could not describe her location. Operators began to trace the call, but suddenly, there was silence. When police reached the desperate teenager, she lay dead in the phone booth, the receiver clutched in her hand.

I have shared these two examples from our hot line files to illustrate the need so many pregnant young girls and women have for crisis telephone counseling. At this moment there are literally thousands of them across the country who feel totally isolated during their time of crisis. Right now they are praying for someone who will help them escape the terror that surrounds them. Most of the calls we handle are from those who are in desperate need of immediate help.

Through the Godparent Centers thousands of callers have been placed in our shepherding homes in Lynchburg or around the country. Hundreds of babies have been saved and placed with qualified Christian families who have been waiting, praying, and hoping to find a baby. Thus these thousands of mothers have found help and hope in Christ through the Christian workers who share their time, their homes, their skills, and their own personal faith. Although some of the stories end tragically, most of them illustrate how young lives can be rescued from misery and despair.

Phase One succeeded all too well. The crisis hot line uncovered tens of thousands of young women across the country who desperately needed and wanted services from

Liberty Godparent Homes. However, volunteer shepherding homes could not provide adequate care for the underaged pregnant girls who were calling for help. Unwed pregnant teenagers, like Jennifer, needed twenty-four hour care and counsel and supervision. They needed to continue or complete their schooling. They needed friends of their own age as company during the difficult time of separation from their families.

Close to 1.1 million of the women becoming pregnant in 1982 were teenagers or younger with more than half a million of them deciding to kill their babies because they didn't feel they had another choice. Godparent Center hot lines were handling thousands of calls from those girls every week. Even after referring these young girls to every available Christian agency like our own, it was impossible to meet the huge demand for assistance to save all these babies. Out of that need for safe, happy, Christian places where young girls could go to live during their pregnancies, we began to plan for Liberty Godparent maternity homes across the nation, reaching out to tens of thousands of young pregnant girls with just the kind of help they desired.

We decided to start with one Liberty Godparent Home in Lynchburg where we could try out our ideas. When we had perfected the plan, we would launch the Phase Two maternity homes in towns and cities across the nation.

In order to begin Phase Two, we needed a large home in a neighborhood not far from Thomas Road Baptist Church. Those of us who had been working with the pregnant girls knew how important that home would be. The girls would come to us scared and lonely. They would be separated from their family and friends (most of them away from home for the first time) for the remaining months of their pregnancy. We wanted a house that would feel like home, but would still house fifteen to twenty girls, twenty-four hour live-in dorm "parents" and "grandparents," the counseling and medical staff, a clinic, necessary administrative support offices, and the emergency telephone hot line center. We searched every neighborhood in Lynchburg for that perfect house. Unfortunately we couldn't afford what we needed, and what we could afford we didn't think good enough for the girls we would serve.

Then one Friday afternoon, David Fleming, our first administrator of Liberty Godparent Ministries and one of my staff at Thomas Road Baptist Church, called from a pay phone in downtown Lynchburg.

"Jerry, come quick!" he exclaimed, his voice full of excitement. "I've found the house we need."

The staff involved in this project jumped into my four-wheel-drive truck and drove from Thomas Road Baptist Church to the historic former Florence Crittenden home on Eldon Street. The rambling, two-story white frame house sat in a tree-lined neighborhood of old Lynchburg that had later operated from 1977 to 1982 as a home for emotionally disturbed teenagers. In March of 1982 the home had been closed for lack of funds.

Some of you might remember a Florence Crittenden home in your town or city. They were founded as biblically based, Christian service centers ministering to the nation's unwed teenage mothers for nearly a century. First the pill and then abortion limited the number of pregnant girls needing help. Little by little many of the centers dropped their Christian emphasis in order to obtain state and federal funding to keep their doors open. And though each of the Florence Crittenden centers had its own history, many of the centers, cut off from their original spiritual roots, simply atrophied and died.

The Victorian house, replete with gables, turrets, and paint-flaked gingerbread trim, sat in a quiet, middle-class neighborhood. A two-story dormitory wing had been added and two oversized trailers on property nearby had been used as classrooms. There was space for almost everything we needed.

The cement block dorm rooms were austere, but they faced a beautiful yard and were shaded by lovely old oak trees. Paint, curtains, and pictures on those whitewashed walls would eliminate the interior drabness. A large, functional kitchen and two spacious dining rooms could feed the young women, live-in staff, and visitors conveniently. A small but adequate medical clinic would meet our prenatal and maternity care needs. The first floor of the dormitory wing could provide offices for the staff. In short, the house was perfect, a gift from God.

Three major obstacles had to be overcome before we could dedicate that magnificent property for our maternity home ministry. First, we had to buy it, and that wouldn't be easy. Our church budget had been committed for the year. It was difficult enough to pay for the Phase One operation for our Liberty Godparent Ministries, but to find another $300,000 in start-up funds for Phase Two was a Herculean task. Second, we had to get a state license to run a maternity home in that beautiful old house and we had no idea if the state would approve one owned and operated by a Christian church. Third, we had to find a Christian social worker and an administrator for the program who were committed to our dream and had the qualifications and experience to help us see the dream come true in Lynchburg and across the country.

Is There a Better Way?

A realtor in our church brought us the first bad news.

"The city's latest tax assessment on the building and the property of the old Crittenden home is $273,000," he said, looking away to avoid seeing the disappointment each of my staff felt as that huge figure was announced. Where would we get a quarter of a million dollars to buy a home that was just the first expensive step in building Phase Two of the program?

"But," he added hopefully, "at current market prices, I appraise the real value at about $150,000." Though that figure was more reasonable, it was still a lot of money to my staff and the Liberty Godparent Ministries volunteers. When the Florence Crittenden board of directors learned of our interest, they invited me to a board meeting to discuss the home and our dreams for it. We didn't know which figure the board would present as their price for the building. We had decided that we could afford to offer $80,000 for the building with a downpayment of $32,000, the rest to be paid in five equal increments over the next five years.

The board met in the old game room of the now-abandoned center, which had been a smoking lounge for the emotionally handicapped teenagers. Old chairs were grouped around a pool table. The walls needed paint. The floors were stained. The carpets were frayed. The home was going into default. These board members had volunteered their time and their money to help the work of the Florence Crittenden center because they cared for teenagers. When I told them our dream for a Liberty Godparent Home, they listened carefully, making notes, asking questions, and looking through the documentation of what the Godparent Centers had accomplished in the past six months through the hot line, the counseling services, and the shepherding homes.

"Thank you, Reverend Falwell," they finally said after my presentation. "We'll let you know."

I left that meeting determined that this stately old home would not end up another victim of the wrecker's ball. I promised myself that no shopping center or condominium development would stand on this spot if I could help it. The girls needed a place like this. They would be driven up to the home surrounded by green lawns and colorful flower beds. Dorm parents would meet the girls and show them to their rooms looking out over old Lynchburg. Beginning at that moment the girls would feel that their home away from home was more than just a dormitory. It would be a symbol of hope that would stand forever.

Why this attention to aesthetic detail? We know that an unwanted pregnancy makes a teenage girl feel ugly, embarrassed, and unwanted. Discovering herself pregnant often causes her self-esteem to nosedive. The young woman feels like hiding her shame from the world. She may even think of death because of that unwanted life growing within her. That's why it becomes so easy to kill the baby, to end the nightmare, and to try to begin again. That's why Liberty Godparent maternity homes provide a sense of permanence, safety and beauty to restore self-confidence and self-worth in the pregnant girls it exists to serve.

Time passed. We waited and prayed and worried. Others began bidding for the property. Real estate developers made plans to build on this parcel of land immediately adjacent to a prime business area of Lynchburg. We knew that almost anyone could outbid our meager offer.

Then, suddenly, the call came. The Crittenden board had decided to sell us the entire property—lock, stock, and barrel—for the $80,000 we had offered. In a newspaper story

the next day, Clay Chapman, president of the board explained why. "We didn't want to see that great old property
become a hot dog stand," he told a reporter. "We preferred
that it continue offering human services."

We thanked God that day for the miracle of obtaining that
beautiful old house. It was a confirmation of our desire to
save unborn lives. Our staff and volunteers walked through
it like a young couple looking over their first home. We
dreamed of the lives that would be changed there. We
planned schedules and made deadlines. We prayed over
every single room. Although we had only three girls in
shepherding homes in Lynchburg at the time—one each
from Ohio, North Carolina, and Virginia—we dreamed of
the day not far off when this first maternity home would
have eighteen to twenty girls, a complete staff, and a hot
line center with calls pouring in from around the nation. It
would be the first maternity center in a family of centers
throughout the nation.

That left only two obstacles between the dream of a Liberty Godparent maternity home for young women and the
realization of that dream. The home would have to be licensed by the state of Virginia and a director, suitable to the
state and to our own goals, would have to be found. Volunteers were mobilized to bring the old home up to the current state safety standards, and my staff and I began the long
and tiring search to find a director for the maternity home.
We read dozens of resumes from men and women all
across the country who applied for the position.

The state of Virginia requires a master's degree in social
sciences and five years of social work experience to qualify
for the position of executive director of a dual program, like
Liberty Godparent Ministries, which has both a maternity

home and an adoption agency. We added to those requirements a commitment to Christ and His church, evidence of
an exemplary Christian lifestyle, and experience in Christian ministry. Finding that director became another example of God's ability to provide just what we needed at the
exact time and place we needed him. Jim Savley, a staff
member who was helping in the search, and I discussed
more than one hundred resumes without finding the person we needed to fill the job. Then one Friday, Jim put his
own resume down before me.

"I think I'm your man," he said smiling sheepishly.

I picked up the file but I already knew its contents well. I
wondered why I hadn't thought of it first. Jim Savley had a
master's degree in the social sciences. He was an expolice-
man who had been the director of undercover narcotics op-
erations for a district attorney's office in Tennessee. He had
worked for several years in a drug rehabilitation program for
adolescents who suffered from drug addiction and sub-
stance abuse. He had taught classes on the danger of drug
misuse in the public schools. At the same time he had been
elected alderman for White House, a satellite community
of Nashville. He had been on the board of directors of a re-
tirement community and the department of parks and rec-
reations there.

Meanwhile as he worked to serve his community, God
had called Jim Savley into full-time Christian ministry. He
had commuted from his home to finish seminary training at
Liberty Seminary, another educational ministry of the
Thomas Road Baptist Church. He pastored a little church in
South Boston, Virginia, while completing his biblical training. When I first shared my dream for the Liberty Godparent Ministries on our weekly television program, Jim had

approached his own congregation to begin Phase One of the program. He and his people had started a hot line in South Boston and were offering callers the opportunity to live in shepherding homes of volunteers in the congregation. When I had hired Jim Savley to my staff, I wasn't searching for a director of a maternity home.

I share this story just in case you are part of a community or church that is considering a Phase One or Phase Two Godparent ministry of your own. Don't be afraid of the standards set by your city or state. You will be amazed at the people whom God has prepared to meet and exceed those standards. It could be that they are already sitting in the pews of your church, just praying for a chance to minister.

When we applied for our maternity home license, our church leaders didn't know what to expect. Would our obvious commitment to creating a Christian environment for the young women disqualify us from licensure? Would our rules of behavior for the proposed home be too "religious" to be acceptable? Would our conservative reputation make us suspect to the decision makers in a state government bureaucracy? We worried, but we worried needlessly.

Within a few short weeks our license was granted. State officials welcomed our maternity program with open arms. They were staggered by the inability of the public sector to meet this need and welcomed help from the private, religious sector. In July 1982, we began Phase Two of the Liberty Godparent Ministries, a maternity home where underaged women could find a sanctuary to save their babies from the horror of abortion.

Just days later we completed renovations of the old Crittenden mansion and moved the crisis phone lines into our new home on Eldon Street. Jim Savley and his small staff set up their offices. Curtains were hung and used furniture was placed in the dormitory rooms. A donated relic of a piano was tuned by a volunteer from the Thomas Road Baptist Church choir and new study Bibles designed for young people, new hymnbooks complete with a section of upbeat Gospel songs and choruses, and a whole collection of donated Christian literature was uncrated and shelved. Medical supplies were purchased by our part-time nurse and a small clinic was made ready for our first admission.

Although Jennifer was one of our early guests at the Liberty Godparent's Home, she was not the first. Tammy, fourteen years old and five months pregnant, was the first young woman we served. She and her mother came to Lynchburg on the very day Tammy's abortion had been scheduled.

"Could I get a drink of water?" she asked, her voice barely above a whisper. Tammy sat awkwardly in a used secretary's chair that had been donated by a local merchant, her fingers locked together supporting her already swollen abdomen. She and her mother were going through the first stages of admission.

Obviously hot and miserable from her day-long drive from the nation's capital and from the stressful process that had led to her journey to Lynchburg, Tammy accepted the glass of water gratefully and gulped it down in one long swallow.

"We were supposed to be in New York today," the young girl said, wiping her lips with the back of one hand. "I was going to get an abortion."

In the state of Virginia, a late second trimester abortion is illegal except in special circumstances. Nevertheless, in many states, such as New York, an abortion is easy to obtain almost to the day of the baby's scheduled delivery. For someone like Tammy to travel to a distant, more permissive state for a late-term abortion is very common. Unfortunately, 44 percent of abortions done after the twenty-first week of gestation are performed on young girls. Like Tammy, many unwed teenage girls don't realize or refuse to believe that they are pregnant until they feel the baby kicking.

There are doctors and clinics across the nation who specialize in late-term abortions. Their most common method for killing the child is through the instillation of prostaglandins, the chemical that cuts off the oxygen supply to the fetus and literally strangles the unborn baby to death. Other abortionists, in order to prevent "the unfortunate occurrence of live birth," use the knife-and-suction method to cut the child from the uterine wall, slice the unborn baby into fragments, and then suction those fragments from the mother's womb.

Last year in Wichita, Kansas, a doctor who specialized in late-term abortions was arrested for selling the infants his abortion patients thought were dead. Apparently the doctor delivered the unborn child by Caesarean section, and while the mother recuperated, the infant was sold on the black market to the highest bidder. The doctor was arrested and the black market baby ring broken up when he tried to sell an "aborted" child to an undercover police officer and his wife for $60,000.

Tammy and her mother had decided to go to New York for a late-term abortion. Her mother, who worked in a federal governmental office, heard about the Godparent Center hot line and called for advice about her daughter. We rushed her a packet of materials explaining the dangers of abortion and offering her the services of the program. Tammy and her mother drove to Lynchburg and sat down with Jim Savley to go through the materials further.

"When I showed Tammy the pictures of an unborn child at five months," Jim told me later, "she wept."

"Look, Mommy," she said, pointing at the pictures, "the baby has hands and feet and eyes. How could we kill it?"

Of course it is a risk to sit down with a fourteen-year-old girl like Tammy who is already five months pregnant and tell her the consequences of abortion, because that new information raises again the very difficult dilemma for the unwed mother and her family. On the surface it seems easier to pay for an abortion than go through the pain, expense, and embarrassment of letting the unborn child go full term to take his or her place in the world. Nevertheless, it has been our experience that short-term discomfort leads to long-term physical and mental health for a young mother and to the saving of the life of that mother's baby. Tammy and her mother sat quietly as they considered Jim Savley's words. Suddenly, Tammy looked at her watch and began to weep quietly.

"It's one o'clock," she said. "My baby would be dead now if we had gone to New York."

Then Tammy looked into her mother's eyes and silently begged for permission to stay at the Godparent Home for the duration of her pregnancy.

For a long moment Tammy's mother stood with her hands at her side as if looking across the distance the unwanted pregnancy had created between them. Then slowly she reached out to Tammy, took her daughter in her arms, and said quietly, "Everything will be all right, darling. Everything will be all right now."

Imagine Tammy's predicament. Fourteen years old and five months pregnant, she was away from home for the very first time and living in a spacious but almost empty old house. There were plenty of people around but all of them were strangers. Jim and his staff were housed on the first floor of the dorm wing. There were two newly trained single women who lived in the dormitory and two sets of group parents who lived in the house apartment. Besides the full-time, twenty-four hour a day staffers, there was a part-time nurse, a cook, and a chaplain present during the daylight hours. However, it didn't take long for Tammy to warm up to the crowd of strangers who showered their love and God's love on her so lavishly.

And though there was already a list of young girls waiting to be admitted, Jim and his staff decided to admit the applicant girls over a period of several months rather than fill up the house immediately. There was so much to be learned about running an effective maternity home and so little time in which to learn it.

During the first week Tammy was given a battery of psychological tests by a social worker. A doctor and a nurse began to compile a complete medical record and a profile of her pregnancy. She was tested and treated for any communicable disease she might be carrying. (Sometimes we forget that gonorrhea, syphilus, and other venereal diseases are epidemic in our country's teenage population, including junior high and elementary school children.) An educational counselor gave her basic skills tests. Then, the professional staff reviewed Tammy's file to determine if our program was appropriate for her needs.

Both Tammy and Jennifer learned at intake that there are four basic rules at Liberty Godparent Homes, and the guest must agree to abide by those rules while she is with us. First, the girls cannot drink alcoholic beverages or use "recreational" drugs. That isn't just a "typical Fundamentalist hangup," as one critic claimed; we are working to save unborn babies, and drug and alcohol use are counterproductive to the health of the baby and of the mother. Second, there is no dating while the pregnant girl is in the program. Third, she must agree to keep all counseling, classroom, or medical appointments that she makes or that are made for her. Fourth, she will attend church regularly on her Sundays in Lynchburg.

An applicant is admitted after her basic screening is complete and she agrees to abide by the house rules. Minors are assigned a single or shared room in our maternity home. Older girls are assigned to a shepherding home. Sometimes, when there is no shepherding home immediately available, an older girl is housed temporarily at the maternity home, but in most cases minors live at the Godparent Home and mature, adult women stay in private, volunteer shepherding homes throughout the city.

After they've had time to move in and get settled, our girls are given a daily schedule and a personal handbook to guide them in the program. They are assigned to licensed counselors and are told their weekly therapy time. Each is given the opportunity to complete requirements for a high school diploma and to sign up for various electives in practical arts, skill development programs, and the various craft classes taught by our volunteers. She is assigned a "big sister" who invariably becomes an important friend and ally during the months of pregnancy. She begins her prenatal care and Lamaze delivery classes immediately.

If all of this sounds like a heavy load, it is. The girls are not in the program simply to relax and have their babies. They are being shaped by our staff and volunteers into productive, mature Christian women able to face the difficult and demanding responsibilities that lie ahead. While they are being trained in office and classroom they also get experience in the field as well. Mature women get part-time or full-time jobs to which they commute daily from their shepherding homes.

Younger girls learn basic child-rearing and homemaking skills. Because they are encouraged not to make their final decision regarding the baby's future until their eighth month of pregnancy, the young women must be equipped to care for their babies if they do not place them for adoption. They go to the stores and learn about Infamil and Similac, about Pampers and Huggies, about baby foods and medicines. Each person also begins an individualized spiritual growth program called Prime-Time, which helps to develop spiritual muscle in addition to the physical and psychological muscles she is building.

The days are full. There is often a chorus of groans and complaints when the alarm clocks go off and another busy day begins. But discipline is necessary. There is much to learn and so little time to learn it. Because of their unwanted pregnancy, these girls must become women overnight. Because of an irresponsible sexual act, whether forced or intentional, they are catapulted out of childhood into a world of adult knowledge and responsibilities. This premature aging takes place if an abortion is performed or if the pregnancy is allowed to take its course, although having an abortion often causes the transition to be ignored. But, we feel that it is our task to help make an effective crossing from one world into the other. For a fourteen-year-old girl like Tammy it can be a lonely and frightening time. However, now when Tammy looks back on those months at Liberty Godparent Home, she smiles with gratitude and praise for what the staff and volunteers did for her and for her baby.

"It wasn't easy," she remembers. "I was really scared when I arrived. But the people at the home loved me, and when I look back on all they did for me in such a short time, I can't believe it. They got me ready for life in four short months. I couldn't have made it without them."

As our very first guest, Tammy had her pick of the dormitory rooms, and the staff helped her decorate it with her own teenage choice of posters, a collection of stuffed animals, and even brightly colored wallpaper to match her bedspread and curtains. Those first lonely nights in the empty dormitory, Tammy lay on her bed clutching a stuffed teddy bear only long enough to be sure that the group parents were in their rooms. Then she tiptoed down the stairs and curled up on Grandma and Grampa Cook's sofa to watch television and eat popcorn until she fell asleep. Grampa Cook has been "Gramps" to more than a hundred young women since he and Mrs. Cook moved into the Liberty Godparent Home, yet he remembers Tammy well.

The Cooks are just two members of our professional child care staff who are available to the girls twenty-four hours a day. We process each group parent carefully. Each comes highly recommended. Each is carefully trained. Each offers his or her own unique personality traits and spiritual gifts in the service of these young girls in need. Almost immediately, the girls adopt the group parents as surrogate parents or grandparents of their own. For many of our young guests, it is the first time they have known genuine, undemanding love from anyone. Many of our youngest girls are victims of incest. Their dads, their brothers, their uncles, even their grandfathers have made them pregnant. They are naturally and wisely suspicious of every man in their lives, so it takes time for group parents to demonstrate that real love exists and that they won't be tricked or trapped or betrayed by it.

Four weeks before her delivery, Tammy had to make the second most difficult decision of her life. Our counseling staff agreed that adoption in Tammy's case was the preferred option. Tammy and her mother disagreed. Tammy kept her baby.

It is difficult for me to explain what really happens to the pregnant girls who go through our maternity program. One has to experience life at 520 Eldon Street to really understand it. That's why Jennifer's story is so important. That's why I've asked her to share it with you.

7
A Surprising Friday the Thirteenth

JENNIFER

I had packed my suitcase and zipped up my hanging bag. Dad had the car in the driveway with the motor running. Mom stood in the doorway of my room waiting.

For a moment she watched me staring at my wall of pictures. Most of them were of Jeff or of Jeff and me on the beach, at the senior prom, or at graduation in our caps and gowns. We had taken three candids in one of those little photo booths at the state fair, with me sitting in Jeff's lap while he made faces over my shoulder.

I had taken most of the pictures down before it hit me. I was going away to have Jeff's baby but there had been no engagement, no bridal showers, no wedding ring. There would be no marriage. There would be no first apartment. No family. There would be a baby but I would have the baby alone in a maternity home in Lynchburg, Virginia. One last picture of Jeff smiled down at me. I pulled it from the wall and placed it in the wastebasket with the others. My dreams for so many things seemed to end up in the wastebasket that day. I didn't cry or feel angry. I just felt numb and tired and very, very sad for what might have been.

Then Mom said, "I'll carry your makeup kit." She was smiling a courageous little smile. "Is the hanging bag ready?" She bustled about my room, filling her arms with things I was taking to the maternity home, and headed down the stairway. Her eyes were damp and her lip trembled as she tried to hide her feelings, just as I was trying to hide mine.

I suppose she felt her dreams were dying too. I was supposed to be going away to college. Instead, I was going away to a maternity home to have a baby. It was disappointing and embarrassing and frightening all at the same time.

We traveled those ten hours to Lynchburg without talking much. Each of us had a picture of what the Liberty Godparent Home would look like. Each of us wondered what would happen to me there. As we neared the historic little town, we drove through gentle hills on iron-red clay, blanketed by deep green forests. The sky was azure blue and great white clouds piled up over the Blue Ridge Mountains. We followed the road past a new shopping center and an historic old red brick church, and then wound our way on a tree-lined street through a gentle neighborhood of old but tidy homes, with neat lawns and front porches with swings.

Dad drove our car into the long circular driveway at 520 Eldon Street and we sat looking up at my temporary new home.

"It's big," he said.

"It's beautiful," my mom chimed in enthusiastically.

"It's old," I said, remembering my visions of a haunted house and a hunchback nurse in army boots. Then I noticed two squirrels playing at the base of a giant oak tree and a noisy bluejay scolding them from a branch overhead. Two very pregnant girls were sitting on a bench nearby feeding bread crumbs to a flock of sparrows that darted about them. There were green lawns and bright yellow flowers. It was Friday the thirteenth but nothing seemed quite so ominous as it had before.

Dad opened the door for me. Mom hurried to help me with the luggage. They were trying hard to make this moment easy. Dad held my hand as we walked into the tiny entry hall in the office wing of that grand old house.

"Mr. Savley told me to bring you right in," the receptionist said cheerily as she led us around the corner and down a hallway filled with tiny offices to meet the director, Jim Savley.

"You must be Jennifer" he said, coming around the desk to greet me. "Welcome to Lynchburg."

I liked him right away because he talked to me first, as though I was the most important person in the room. He was round-faced and pleasant. There were pictures on the wall of his wife and family. Near me I could see a framed telegram from President Reagan, a few certificates and diplomas, and an impressive painting of Mary riding on a donkey carrying the baby Jesus in her arms. Joseph walked close by. They were traveling through a desert on a journey somewhere. I tried to remember the story, but all I could see was the look in Mary's eyes as she stared lovingly into her baby's face.

"Do you like the painting, Jennifer?" Jim Savley was sitting on the edge of his desk looking down at me. "Mary and Joseph are fleeing to Egypt to save the life of their baby," he said.

I understood why the painting was chosen for his office. My family and I had traveled to Lynchburg for a similar reason—to save my baby. There was an unborn child growing inside me and this time that baby would not die.

The LGH director spent the next half hour explaining why the program was founded. "There are lots of places that provide what they call 'an alternative to pregnancy,' " he said. "We provide what we call 'an alternative to abortion.' "

Apparently he already knew the history of my first pregnancy. I felt embarrassed about the abortion. I felt doubly embarrassed about being pregnant again. I had been so smug and determined when I left the Planned Parenthood office after my abortion two years before. I thought kids who got pregnant were losers or victims or both. And I was certain that kids who got pregnant the second time were really out of it. I thought it wasn't possible for me to get pregnant again.

After all, I had thought to myself proudly, I was a Christian. I was part of the youth group at church. I was a straight A student with a "senior superlative" rating, an honor reserved for people at the top of the graduating class. After my junior high years of awkward ugliness, I had even been voted "Best Looking" by my fellow students. I had loving parents and a lot of good friends. My future was secure. I could have what I wanted out of life. I would never end up having a baby in a maternity home hidden away in a tiny town in Virginia. I was certain of it, but I was wrong again. And worst of all, this time I had no one to blame but myself.

"Many of the girls at the home have had abortions before," Mr. Savley informed me. "Just like you had, Jennifer. We don't look down on them for what they did or didn't do

126

in the past. We are glad that they have found the courage to do the right thing now. And we are here to help them do it in every way we can."

There were rules to be read, forms to sign, schedules to learn, and self-improvement programs to understand. I went through those first stages of admission in a daze. My parents asked questions. Mr. Savley answered them. I hardly heard a word. I just stared at the painting of Mary looking into the face of the baby she was trying to save and thought about the baby growing inside me.

"Well, how about a tour?" Jim asked and I looked up quickly and nodded. It was about the last thing I really wanted. Before arriving in Lynchburg I had pictured the worst. Monastic cells. Long, dark, shadowy corridors with bats and cobwebs. And, of course, a dungeon.

"This is one of our two dining rooms," Jim said proudly as he led Mom and Dad and me into a small room with a bay window overlooking the garden. Early American maple tables and chairs were arranged to seat the girls and their room parents in small groups of five or six.

"And this is our chef," Jim added as he took a large bag of groceries from a young woman just entering the dining room, her arms filled with packages and parcels of food.

"Sharon," he said, and then nodded in my direction, "this is Jennifer Simpson and her parents."

Sharon smiled broadly and led us into the kitchen. She was only twenty-four, the wife of a Liberty University student. She was small and quiet, and both Mom and I were drawn to her immediately. Sharon was proud of her kitchen and what she accomplished for the girls there. The refrigerators were oversized and the stove was black and huge, but everything else looked like home. Mom bustled about after

Sharon. They unloaded grocery sacks of corn on the cob, iceberg lettuce, carrots, and honeydew melons. They talked about menus and natural foods and vitamins important to my baby.

"Jennifer loves apple crisp and ice cream," my mother whispered to Sharon confidentially, "but she needs help with broccoli and spinach."

I was about to defend my eating habits when I noticed my mother lean heavily against a long kitchen counter and turn her face away from us. Sharon walked immediately to my mother's side and put one arm around her. My dad turned away. I watched them both fight back their tears and loved them more than I had ever loved them.

We continued our tour through the rooms filled with old but well-kept furniture, lamps, books, and games. We passed the hot line center where an operator was counseling on the toll-free pregnancy crisis line. We peeked into Grampa and Grandma Cook's apartment downstairs, the laundry room, and the sundry closet, where girls could get a few supplies and late night "munchies."

"Why don't we go upstairs and move you in," Jim finally suggested after we had completed our tour of the entire downstairs area of 520 Eldon Street. I knew that the moment I placed my foot on that bottom stair, the countdown would begin for my parents to leave me in that place. I wanted to see my room but I didn't want my parents to leave. Just days before I had been glad to be rid of them. Now, I wanted them around forever.

"Normally you would be staying in a shepherding home," Jim said as we walked up the stairs behind him. "Girls who have graduated from high school shouldn't really need the disciplines and routine of the maternity home. But all of our homes are full and there won't be any available for a while," he explained. "So, until we find one for you, you'll share this three-bed room with two other girls in our program."

Dad placed my cases on the one empty bed. Mom opened my hanging bag and began to place my winter clothing in the closet. My roommates had already gone to the Thomas Road Baptist Church for an evening Bible study. They had left the room neatly cluttered with teddy bears and other favored dolls and stuffed animals, hair dryers, books, and magazines. Both girls had pictures of boys on their dressers. I thought of Jeff and the pictures I had thrown away.

Mom nudged the mattress firmly with the heel of her hand. She picked up a corner of the quilt and whispered to herself, "Look at this beautiful handmade quilt." She smoothed down one corner of the quilt and fluffed my pillow. "Some dear soul made one for every bed."

Jim Savley was the first to leave. "I've an appointment," he said. "Call me any time of the day or night if you have questions. Remember, we'll take good care of your daughter. You have nothing at all to worry about."

Then, without another word, he was gone. Dad stood on one side of my bed looking at me. Mother stood at the other. We had cried enough tears. It was time to say good-bye.

"Call us, Jen," my father said hugging me and swallowing hard. "Take good care of our baby," Mom added proudly.

They closed the tall white door behind them. I could hear them walking slowly down the steps. I heard the firedoor slam behind them. I walked quickly to the window and watched them walking hand-in-hand back to our car. Dad opened the door for Mom and then looked up in the direction of my room. I waved and smiled down at them. They were both staring up at me. Dad waved back. Then they drove away quickly and I stood there looking down at the empty driveway long after they had gone.

I unpacked my suitcases and filled the drawers of the little bureau near my bed. Though it was still early evening I got into my pajamas, crawled under the covers, tucked that homemade quilt around me, and lay there looking at my new home.

The walls were off-white cinderblock, the floors were carpeted with low pile shag in shades of green and gray. The dresser next to my bed was oak and several of the knobs on the drawers didn't match. The curtains were a yellow chintz with lots of ruffles.

The quilts on each bed were made of scraps with a white backing and little tufts of yarn tied every eight inches. I noticed that both of my roommates had turned the white backside up, so that from a distance the quilts looked like white bedspreads with a bright green dotted Swiss design.

The bathrooms down the hall were large, with two shower stalls, two sinks, and three lavatories to accommodate comfortably six of us girls. The floors were little hexagons of alternating black-and-white tile, and they were clean but smelled musty with a thin disguise of Lysol. It was an old house, big and comfortable and lived-in.

I awakened my first morning in Lynchburg to the sounds of my two new roommates. I pretended to be asleep, but I watched them both through squinty lids. A tall, blonde girl was bent over double and drying her hair from underneath with a loud hair dryer on blowtorch speed. When she finished, she threw back her head like a wild pony to give her hair that "California look" and proceeded to work styling mousse into the roots. The other girl was seriously over-weight and wore a plaid polyester jumper with knee socks and loafers. She looked poor and frightened and a long way from home. Occasionally, she would steal a look at the blonde or at me and then just as quickly look away again. She held a tube of mascara the way a child holds a crayon and dabbed it on her eyelashes ineffectively.

When the call for breakfast sounded, the larger girl disap-peared quickly without a word. The tall blonde finished perfecting her "look," refusing to be rushed by anyone. Af-ter one last look into the mirror she walked toward the door and without even looking in my direction said, "Don't worry about breakfast. I'll bring up some fruit." Then she was gone.

During the next three months at 520 Eldon, I learned to love those two very different girls and to care about them in ways I've never cared for anyone. Leona was from Alabama. She weighed about eighty pounds more than the nurse al-lowed. It was hard to tell how pregnant Leona was with all the extra weight she carried. One afternoon she came back from her medical checkup all excited about losing three pounds on her "food only" diet. She rushed into the room, plopped down on the edge of my bed to share her good news, and promptly broke and collapsed the bed under both of us. We called her "Big Mama" after that. She was the daughter of a Baptist preacher in a southern mountain town.

Kaye was quite a different story. She was a beautiful girl with an ugly past. Her parents lived in Reno, Nevada. She had been physically abused by her natural father and sexu-ally molested by her stepdad. Her mother had been very beautiful and very dumb. Kaye had her first abortion when she was fifteen. She didn't like to talk about her past. At first she seemed aloof and arrogant. It was just a cover. She had been hurt so many times by so many people, she was afraid of being hurt again.

Missy was fourteen and roomed with Gail in the two-bed room next to ours. Missy was eight months pregnant and hungry all the time. Every night after the lights were out and the last giggles quieted, Missy would walk the halls repeating her midnight litany, "Anybody got an extra granola bar?"

Missy's roommate, Gail, was older than Missy but equally pregnant. She was cool under pressure and mothered us all during our times of crisis and panic. The staff trained Gail to answer the pregnancy hot line. She was very good working with girls from around the country who called in with problems that Gail had experienced first-hand.

"Gail!" Missy yelled from the bottom of the stairs in the middle of one night, "You're wanted on the hot line."

It was almost 2:00 A.M. The hot lines are answered twenty-four hours a day by trained people, and Missy had walked into the phone center on her late night hunger mission when a suicide call had been received. The caller had given her name and asked specifically for Gail. Missy had been sent to retrieve her roommate.

"It's that girl in Ohio again," Missy yelled so that everyone on both floors could hear it. "She's committing suicide. You've got to save her."

Missy was really into this one. I could hear Gail getting out of bed. She walked sleepily across her room and opened the door. Missy screamed again. "Hurry, Gail," she called frantically, " 'Ohio' will die before you get there."

Gail got to the top of the stairs and looked down at her distraught roommate. "Tell 'Ohio,' " she said quietly, "to take two aspirin with a glass of orange juice, get a good night's sleep, and call me in the morning."

"But she'll be dead," Missy gasped. "And you'll have killed her."

"That's all right," she answered, turning from the emergency and plodding slowly back to her room. "Then I'll take the aspirin with the orange juice and I'll get a good night's sleep."

"Gail!" Missy called one last time.

"Night, Missy," Gail answered, knowing exactly what she was doing. She'd dealt with "Ohio" enough times before to know that her threats were nothing more than...a bluff.

Of course Missy was beside herself. "You've killed her," she said coming back to her room after delivering Gail's message. "Does anybody have a granola bar?" she added, poking her head into our room and groaning hungrily.

In fact, Gail was an expert in knowing when a crisis was real and when it wasn't. She succeeded very well with her caller from Ohio. The girl arrived at Liberty Godparent Home three weeks later, much to Missy's relief. But the night of her call, Missy thought the girl had killed herself for sure. Missy couldn't sleep for worrying. In fact, she ended up in our room that night sitting in the middle of our floor eating every little snack Leona had stored away and muttering about that "poor little girl in Ohio." The whole scene struck me funny. I laughed until I cried. As I lay on my side teasing Missy and laughing, I felt my baby kick for the very first time.

"Feel!" I said to Kaye who rushed to touch my abdomen, which barely showed any sign of pregnancy.

"Yes, I feel it," she answered.

Leona was there seconds later. "I can feel it, too," she said.

"Let me feel," Missy added, feeling my tummy with one hand and clutching a granola bar in the other.

The three of them had been feeling life within themselves for many weeks. Now I knew for certain that a tiny person with arms and legs, hands and feet was growing inside of me. Suddenly, I wasn't laughing anymore. I was crying and no one could console me.

"What's the matter, Jennifer?" Leona asked, sitting carefully on the edge of my bed.

Kaye knelt beside me and stroked my hair. "It's OK, Jennifer. Go ahead and cry," she said. "It'll do you good."

"She's crying about that poor dead kid up in Ohio," Missy explained as she sat on the floor looking up at me.

"No," Kaye argued, "she's crying for the little live kid growing down inside her."

Kaye was right. I was crying because those little kicks and jabs that I was feeling for the first time were final proof of that living person. All those pictures of unborn babies that I had seen in the maternity care classes and in the reading room were finally real to me. At last I could close my eyes and picture in my womb a little person with his or her eyes closed swimming in his amniotic sac getting life from me. And so I cried.

But Kaye could not know the other reason I was crying. For the first time I had to admit that I had also killed another baby during my abortion. I had never felt that first baby kick or jab inside me. I had never pictured his or her tiny arms or legs, hands or feet, fingers or toes. I hadn't realized—or I couldn't admit—that it was even a baby. I really believed that it was just a mass of sperm and eggs. So I had it cut away, suctioned up, and disposed of. That night, surrounded by my new friends, I really understood what I'd done. I cried for the living baby growing inside me and for the baby that had died.

"Lord, bless Jennifer's baby," said the tiny voice from out of the darkness. I looked up through my tears in the direction of the voice that prayed that four-word prayer.

It was Missy, only thirteen, a girl abused by her father and eight months pregnant by a man she didn't even know. Little Missy trying to complete her junior high classes before she had her baby. Little Missy terminally hungry, still clutching the remains of her midnight snack and worrying about that unknown caller from Ohio. Missy had never prayed before during her three months at LGH. That night she prayed for me.

"And bless our babies, too," she added.

There was a moment of silence. Then in unison Leona and Kaye both said, "Amen." God would bless my baby. I knew it. And He would bless their babies, too. Leona and Kaye both patted my tummy, said "Good night," and crawled back into their beds. I could barely see Missy still sitting there in the darkness. Finally, her snack finished, she stood to leave. At the door Missy turned and whispered to Leona, "You sure you don't have another granola bar?"

Kaye moaned. I laughed again. Leona threw her pillow but Missy was already gone.

During those first weeks at 520 Eldon Street, my attitude had been bitter and resentful. I was disgusted at how fat everyone seemed to get. I hated going to church together on Sundays and Wednesdays because the van would drive right up to the door where everyone could see us, and we would troop out and sit together. One by one, each of the girls would get up to go to the bathroom during the service. The congregation had no doubt about who we were or where we were from.

I remember watching the other girls who were in their eighth and ninth months get "elephant legs" and chubby faces. I determined that I was not going to gain any more weight than I had to. I'd spent the last two years trying to get used to being pretty. I wasn't going to let myself go back to looking frumpy.

I used to lie in bed and stare at the acoustical tile ceiling with the squiggly lines that reminded me of stretch marks. I had vowed not to let it happen to me. I ate only enough to stay alive. Everyone was afraid I'd starve the baby. It didn't matter. I was only eighteen. I didn't want to get stretch marks or to look matronly for the rest of my life.

But everything changed that night I felt my baby moving down inside of me. I had thought only of myself. Suddenly, that little person was the most important thing in the world to me.

My relationship with Mom and Dad also changed during those first months at 520 Eldon Street. Since we weren't able to be with each other, we wrote back and forth almost every day. Even Dad tried to write regularly. It's hard to argue and fight through the mail. Instead those letters and the occasional phone calls drew us close together as a family.

Summer ended. The leaves on the great oak tree outside my window turned gold and brown before they were carried away by cold winds that shuddered and bent the branches. The squirrels darted in and out of their secret places preparing for the winter. The sparrows headed farther south.

Each day I watched Missy and Leona and the others walking across the lawn to their classes in English and math and history. Since I had already finished high school, I worked on special projects, helped Sharon in the kitchen, and wrote letters to my friend, Shelly, and to my parents. I did join the girls for their Lamaze and maternal care classes and for seminars on personal health and budget management. We all attended Sunday worship services and midweek Bible classes together at Thomas Road Baptist Church and our own daily chapel sessions. All eighteen or nineteen girls along with assorted house parents, dorm assistants, nurses, hot line operators, and LGH staff would crowd into the dining rooms and overflow the dining room that had become our chapel. There would be prayers and Bible study, singing, intimate times of sharing, and special guest speakers and discussion leaders.

"Are there any questions?" A young woman professor from Liberty University had just finished an interesting chapel session on developing your prayer life when Missy's hand shot up.

"Do you have any kids, Mrs. Campbell?" Missy asked.

"Why no," our guest answered, looking rather flustered. "I'm not even married."

"Oh, that don't matter," Missy answered, looking around the room. "Who is?"

Needless to say, there was a slight moment of embarrassed silence. Then that chapel session broke up in hysterical laughter that we thought would never end. In fact, Missy's reply—"Oh, that don't matter. Who is?"—became a classic expression around 520 Eldon Street used in every imaginable situation.

The days were long and very full. Besides our daily schedules there were private individual counseling appointments and small group "rap" sessions every week. However, some of the really effective counseling was done informally late at night when we would raid the kitchen. Mr. Cook or Gail would dish out large bowls of mocha almond fudge ice cream to the girls; and as we fed those late night hidden hungers, we let down all the barriers between us. We giggled and we cried. We shared our hopes and our fears for the future. But mainly we talked about having our babies and the hardest decision most of us would ever make: What would we do with our babies once they were born?

"I just know my baby's coming in the next few days," Missy said one evening. She was smiling and pretending to look pleased, but Kaye saw through Missy's bluff.

"So, how does that make you feel," Kaye asked, sitting down beside Missy and spooning a second helping of ice cream into Missy's bowl.

"It makes me feel fine," Missy said with a noticeable quiver in her voice.

"Have you decided about adoption," Kaye asked, noticing that Missy was about to cry.

"I can't give up my baby," Missy said, looking down into her ice cream. "I know I should but I can't."

"Yes, you can," answered a voice from the back of the room.

Missy whirled to face a senior student from Liberty University. Rosemary had been volunteering on the hot line graveyard shift for the past three weeks. Her father was a Christian celebrity. Occasionally Rosemary sat in the back of the dining room during her break and listened to us talk, but until that time she had said nothing.

"How would you know?" Missy asked angrily. "You never had to give a baby away."

"Yes, I did," Rosemary answered. The room grew silent. All of us turned to look at Rosemary with new interest in the story she had never told. Rosemary was a kind of in-house celebrity herself. She was bright and beautiful and talented. She was well-known at Thomas Road Baptist Church for her leadership among the singles. She even taught a very large and very popular high school Bible class that many of us had attended.

"I sat in that very chair, Missy," Rosemary began, "when I was trying to decide about my baby's future." She walked to the empty chair across from Missy and sat down in it.

"I know what it feels like to have a baby inside you kicking and struggling to be born. I know how you grow to love that little person during those nine months she lives inside you. I know the pain of leaving the hospital with empty arms. And I know the awful questions and doubts and guilty feelings you live with after you've given her away."

"So, why do it?" Missy asked. "Why should I do it?"

"You know why, Missy," Rosemary answered. "You love your baby too much to keep her. You don't have a home or a family or a husband to offer your baby. You can't provide anything you want her to have."

Rosemary was telling Missy all those things we wanted her to hear but didn't have the courage to say ourselves. And this time Missy was listening.

"There is," Rosemary continued quietly, "a young couple right this minute who cannot have a baby of their own. They have a good income. They have a beautiful home with a nursery and toys and baby clothes and an empty cradle. They are praying for a baby, Missy. They can take care of the baby. They can give the baby what you want to give her, a home that..."

139

"Stop it," Missy cried. "I want my baby to have a good life. I know I should give her up for adoption. But I'm just not brave enough to do it."

Rosemary reached down and took Missy's hand in hers. "Oh, that doesn't matter," she said quietly. "Who is?"

I lay awake a long time after that trying to make my own decision about adoption. The next morning when the other girls were at class, I decided to discuss the question of adoption with Sharon as we worked together in the kitchen.

Before I had a chance to mention my questions, Sharon exclaimed. "Jennifer, you've popped."

I smoothed my cotton blouse over the bulge where my waist used to be. In the teenage slang of 520 Eldon Street a girl has "popped" when her pregnancy begins to show.

"Do you think it's a bad idea to see your baby afterwards?" I asked her suddenly.

Sharon knew I was troubled. She sat down beside me and we cleaned the broccoli together.

"You've decided to adopt out, haven't you?" Sharon asked already knowing my decision.

It wasn't making the decision that worried me. It was sticking to it.

"Yeah," I answered slowly, "but what about the girls who change their minds when they see their baby for the first time? I don't know if I have the courage to do it."

Sharon really cared about us girls. Like all the personnel at Liberty Godparent Home she had been trained to counsel as well as cook. She didn't talk much. She believed that she ministered to us through her balanced and delicious meals. But often at night or on holidays when the counselors' offices were closed, we used Sharon's kitchen for the counseling room. All the girls liked to mother her four-year-old son, Chad, when his mother brought him along to work.

"I think it's different with different girls," she said. Then looking down at her son playing nearby she added, "I don't think I could have said good-bye without at least seeing him and feeling him in my arms."

"What should I do in the hospital?" I asked. "Should I hold him? Should I feed him? Or should I just look at him through the glass?"

Sharon looked at me and smiled. Her eyes brimmed with tears. She didn't speak at first, but I could tell by the way she looked at me that she understood.

"That is a very important question, Jen," she finally said leaning toward me and taking my hand. "Talk to your counselor about it tomorrow when you see him."

"I will," I promised, "but I want to talk about it to you, too," I said feeling desperate for an answer.

"Do you think the baby will hate me for giving him up?"

"Oh, Jennifer," Sharon answered, "there are so many things we cannot know ahead of time, but we can know this. If you place your baby in love because you think adoption is a better way, then you won't ever have to hate yourself for doing it."

We both sat side-by-side working on the broccoli for a moment. Then she turned to hug me. I could feel her warm tears against my face.

"You know what?" I sobbed. "I still hate broccoli."

Sharon laughed. "But your baby loves it," she added.

Just before noon the very next day, Missy had a seven-pound baby girl. For two days we waited and wondered if she would return alone or with her tiny daughter. Then, Wednesday afternoon, just after lunch, Missy came home to us. Her arms were empty, but she was smiling. We all ran down to greet her.

"She was very beautiful," Missy said as we almost carried her to her room. "She was red and tiny and screaming for granola bars."

Missy lay back on her bed. The room was filled with smiling friends. There were balloons and a "Welcome Home" sign taped to her closet door.

"I held her this morning," she said. "She has brown hair just like mine and pretty blue eyes."

I watched Missy and thought about that day soon when I would hold my own child. Each one in the room was listening to Missy and thinking about the moment when she would stand in Missy's place. We were swallowing hard and sniffling and blinking back our tears as Missy continued.

"She smiled at me," Missy said looking straight up at the ceiling, her eyes brimming with tears. "The nurse said it was gas, but I could see she was really smiling."

For a moment Missy lay there. Then, she sat up on the edge of her bed with a determined look in her eye and a broad smile on her face. "And in just a few days she'll be smiling at her other mommy just like she smiled at me."

The room was filled with pregnant girls looking at Missy and wondering at her courage. Finally, Kaye sat down beside her and took Missy's hands in her own hands and said four short words.

"Lord, bless Missy's baby."

And eighteen girls answered as one, "Amen."

8

Are the Times A-Changing?

JERRY

Last year, in this great land of ours, more than 1.5 million unborn children died before their birthday: silent, helpless, innocent victims of abortion. Remember, while you read this page, at least three babies were aborted in these United States. And during each new page you read, at least three more babies will die. No less than one unborn child dies in his or her mother's womb every twenty seconds, twenty-four hours a day, 365 days a year. The modern world still trembles in horror when it recalls Hitler's murder of more than ten million people in the gas chambers and on the gallows of Dachau, Auschwitz, and Flossenburg during the nightmare of the Nazi Third Reich, but since 1973 more than sixteen million babies have been killed legally by America's doctors with very little public outrage and relatively little public dissent.

That Americans legally murdered so many babies last year is bad enough, but to make the deaths even more senseless, there were five million families who applied to adopt the only fifty thousand babies available. Two million of these families were infertile and unable to have children of their own. These hard statistics come from Dr. Jack Willke, founder and president of the National Right to Life Organization, and from Bill Pierce, president of the National Committee for Adoption.

Liberty Godparent Ministries is working to help right that terrible wrong. Phase Three of our dream is creating and helping others form Christian adoption agencies that work directly with each Liberty Godparent Home across the nation. There may have been only fifty thousand babies available for adoption in 1985, but we believe that truth will conquer the lies about abortion and it will no longer be an acceptable remedy for an unwanted pregnancy.

Already pregnant women across America are beginning to change their minds about abortion. Like Jennifer, they are discovering on their own that the tiny person growing inside them deserves the right to life. In 1985, for the first time in a decade, the abortion rate slowed its climb and began the humane descent back to sanity.

Leaders across the nation are beginning to protest the slaughter of a generation of unborn children. The president has sent a legal brief to the Supreme Court through the attorney general's office requesting that the decision in *Roe* v. *Wade* be overthrown. I believe that it is only a matter of time until abortion is a carefully regulated surgical procedure used only at a time of genuine crisis.

The billion-dollar abortion industry will protest about women's rights. They will fight the pro-life forces, but most abortionists and their clinics are not really interested in women's rights. They are only interested in the six-, or even seven-figure income the abortion boom has guaranteed to so many of them. If they really cared about women's rights, they would read the exhaustive studies by colleagues in their own medical and scientific fields that clearly document the psychological and physical horrors of abortion and its aftermath.

Abortionists have won many battles with their campaign of lies, half truths, and misinformation. But they will lose the war. Liberty Godparent Ministries is gearing up to handle the millions of expectant mothers who want to save their babies and to place them for adoption into qualified, caring homes.

Jennifer has already explained how the program affected her life. She lived for four months in our maternity home in Lynchburg and for another three months in a nearby shepherding home. The Phase One shepherding home experience is normally intended for older girls and women who need emotional support and Christian love during a problem pregnancy and for whom the structure of the maternity home is unnecessary.

A primary reason for writing this book was my hope that people like you who take the time to read it might consider beginning some phase of the program in your town or city. The Liberty Godparent Home in Lynchburg offers a free handbook detailing most of the start-up information you will need and a toll-free line for counseling from our seasoned staff specialists at any point where you might need us.

It is much easier and far less expensive to begin a Phase One operation where you and the volunteers you gather around you offer women in your community emergency care through a crisis hot line, free pregnancy tests, and confidential counseling by Christian doctors, nurses, pastors, and law counselors who volunteer to help. Phase One also includes providing shelters during those months of pregnancy through local shepherding homes. People who volunteer their spare bedroom to an expectant mother provide a vital and demanding contribution to the women the program is dedicated to assist.

The shepherding home experience that Jennifer will describe is a safe shelter for a pregnant girl who has no other viable option. There are two kinds of shepherding homes. The first is simply a home volunteered by a concerned Christian family to provide temporary housing to a young, unwed, pregnant woman who is capable of becoming well-adjusted spiritually, socially, psychologically, and physically. We dare not forget that tens of thousands of Christian girls from stable, loving families find themselves pregnant every year.

These young women may feel scorn and ridicule from their fellow Christians. Their pastors or their Sunday school teachers, their families and Christian friends, may have taken clear stands against abortion but when a young, unmarried woman in church or in a family gets pregnant, these people often do nothing to help. Instead of reaching out to the young woman, instead of helping her understand that her sins, too, can be forgiven and that her baby has a right to live, they make the girl feel so guilty and embarrassed that she ends up like her non-Christian friends—a victim of the abortionist.

These Christian girls need to experience the love of Christ through the love of a caring Christian community. When a church reaches out through a hot line and through shepherding homes to help its own young women and other young women who are in trouble in its community, it can transform that church into one that practices what it preaches. This kind of love in action is a sure guarantee for the multiplication of a church's ministry and growth.

Bonny, a young woman from a rural suburb of Shreveport, Louisiana, is one dramatic example of the positive changes that can happen even during a family's time of crisis. Bonny's father was a pastor of a large evangelical church who asked to see me confidentially at a ministers' meeting where I was speaking. I could tell by the desperate look in his eyes that he needed help right away, so I agreed to meet him in the hotel coffee shop that night after our last session.

He was a rather distinguished looking man in his mid-fifties, well-groomed, articulate, and obviously successful at his profession. But his hands shook. The hot coffee spilled more than once as he held the cup in his trembling hands. He needed time to work up the courage to tell me what was torturing him. I waited, and finally, he spoke.

"I'm in big trouble," he almost whispered, looking over his shoulder to see that none of his colleagues were present to hear what he was about to confess. "My daughter is pregnant." He blurted out the hardest part, "And she isn't married."

I was almost relieved to hear his confession. I had pictured all kinds of horrors that might be tormenting this man. When he said his daughter, a high school graduate, was unwed and pregnant, I breathed a little easier. Don't misunderstand me. This is no small matter. I felt his pain and understood his dilemma. However, over one million fathers in this nation faced a daughter's unwanted pregnancy last year. It is traumatic, it is painful, it is awkward, but it isn't the end of the world. In fact God can bring great good out of this common family tragedy, just as he brought

Solomon from the illegitimate intimacy of David and Bathsheba. Living through a crisis of any kind can cause a family to rediscover Christ's love in and through each other. However, I didn't interrupt; I just listened.

"I'll probably lose my church over this situation," he said suppressing the tears, "and my ministry."

This pastor had preached many sermons on the Christian leader "having his house in order." Apparently, he had criticized and condemned other Christian pastors and laymen privately and in the pulpit for the sins of their families. Now, all the judgment he had loosed on his people was being turned back on him, and he felt the awful weight of it.

"I told her not to date that kid," he said, already beginning to blame someone else for the problems he was facing. "I even took him aside before their first date and made him promise he wouldn't harm my little girl or misuse her in any way."

For the next ten minutes he raged at the nineteen-year-old boy who had made his daughter pregnant. "The boy betrayed me," he said angrily. "I trusted him and he failed me." For a moment my new pastor friend sat staring blankly at the table. Then he continued, "That boy said he was a Christian. His parents were leaders in another church like ours across the city. I thought a Christian boy would never..."

The minister wanted me to believe that his daughter was perfect, blameless, and above reproach. She had been a Christian since the third grade. She was polite, intelligent, creative. She had graduated with honors and was enrolled in her first year in college, where she was studying to be a missionary nurse. The boy, on the other hand, was evil incarnate. As the pastor wound down his angry history, he looked to me for advice. He had seen our television special on Liberty Godparent Ministries called "A Better Way." He wondered if our program could help him and his daughter in this time of crisis.

I've personally admitted only two young women to our LGH program during its entire three-year history. My staff is in charge of that process, but this time, without calling any-one, I invited the pastor to drive his daughter to Lynchburg immediately. I even promised that she would be admitted into a shepherding home without even knowing if we had one currently available.

Looking back, I realize why I took that chance. I felt intui-tively that this desperate pastor was about to get an abor-tion for his daughter. And I was right. The words were never spoken, but I knew that the embarrassment and the anger he felt could easily lead him to a desperate solution. What he couldn't know was the long-term price he would pay for that short-term solution. He was adamantly opposed to abortion—for everyone else. He saw the fetus as a living soul and had preached against the "murder" of the unborn baby, but when he faced the unwanted pregnancy of his own daughter, he wanted the easy way out just like every-body else. There is no easy way out.

That pastor's daughter, Bonny, lived in a shepherding home for the next six months. She told her side of the story to our counseling staff, which I have permission to share with you. I changed her name and her hometown to protect her privacy.

Bonny's boyfriend wasn't the only guilty one in this un-wanted pregnancy. Bonny had found her homelife stifling, and life with her father had been a steady flow of unreasonable demands. She had felt no love from him, only judgment. He pushed her to achieve. He pushed her to perform. He pushed her to take leadership in the church and never seemed satisfied with anything she accomplished. She had gone to her boyfriend for sexual intimacy out of the deep need for the familial intimacy she had never known at home. Little by little Bonny felt her hatred for her father slip away as our community ministered to her and to her unborn baby's needs.

At the same time, Bonny's father was discovering a dimension of love he had never known before. He had preached long and dramatic sermons about Christ's love being demonstrated through the church, but he had never experienced it himself. Upon his return from Lynchburg, he felt obligated to confess his daughter's sin to his board of deacons. He called them together soon after Bonny joined us. He expected them to judge him in the spirit he had judged so many others; instead, they reached out to him. They began to share with him the struggles and failures of their own families. They cried and embraced and asked God's forgiveness and the forgiveness of each other.

Bonny and her father both experienced healing through their family "tragedy." And a young Christian couple who had been waiting for four years to adopt a baby for their own had their dreams come true. When Bonny's father picked her up not long after her delivery of an eight-pound baby boy, they stood in my office with tears running down their faces and confessed the new love they felt for God and for each other.

The shepherding home was perfect for a mature and sensitive young woman like Bonny. But special shepherding homes are often needed to provide shelter to young women who have unusual, sometimes extraordinary, spiritual, social, psychological, or even physical needs. Christian couples or families who volunteer their homes for these unwed mothers are trained by the Liberty Godparent Ministries staff for their task.

The true stories of these needy young women would break your heart. There are hundreds of stories already in our files and thousands of stories in maternity care centers around the nation that should be shared with those trying to take an intelligent and reasonable stand against abortion. It is all too easy to be philosophical about the issue. That the fetus at its earliest stages is a human being is no longer up for debate. That each little unborn child deserves his or her chance at life is no longer a question. That abortion is almost without exception a simple case of murder is all too simple to prove. I will fight the abortionist and his clinic with every ounce of energy I have, but I cannot fight the abortionist without making provisions to care for the young woman who finds herself carrying the unborn child I am fighting to protect.

The pro-life forces, of which I am proudly a part, sometimes err in oversimplifying the issue when it comes to the suffering of the pregnant woman. It is easy for most of us from the safety and comfort of middle class America to look down our noses in judgment at the abortionist and his or her victim. But then we sin as they sin. We must hear and feel the plight of the woman carrying the unborn baby as much as we hear and feel the plight of that unborn child. It didn't take long for me and the people of Thomas Road Baptist Church to realize that we could not take a stand against abortion until we had taken a stand for the mothers of those babies whose right to life we are protecting. Talking to these young women from all across the land has changed my life forever and was the primary reason for founding the program.

JoAnn called the Godparent Center crisis hot line one Saturday at midnight. The operator heard the voice of a frightened fourteen-year-old girl whispering frantically. The words were garbled, and she was obviously terrified.

"Could you speak a bit louder?" the operator inquired. "I'm having trouble hearing you."

"My name is JoAnn," the caller repeated. "I can only talk for a few minutes. My father is drunk and I can hear him snoring, but if he wakes up while I am calling you, he will kill me."

Sensing the girl's urgency, the operator interrupted to get a telephone number or address.

"I can't tell you," the girl answered. "If you show up here, I'm dead."

Suddenly, the caller gasped and the line went dead. The operator was helpless. She waited, hoping the frightened girl would call again. Two hours later after talking to other girls all across the country, the late night crisis counselors got a second call from the same young woman. This time she could share bits and pieces of a real teenage horror story.

"I am fourteen," the girl whispered. "My mother was hurt in a bad car wreck and just stays in bed. She can't move. We have to change her diapers and the bottle that drips food into her arm. She is like a vegetable. After my mom's accident, my daddy started having sex with me. I was eleven. I tried to pretend I was asleep. Sometimes, when my daddy came after me, I got in bed with my mom, but she couldn't help me. Now, I think I'm pregnant. I don't know for sure, but I think I am. How can I find out for sure?"

The operator questioned the girl, trying to get her address, knowing that the appropriate city officials should be notified. The girl was afraid to give her address.

"If you come here, my dad will know I called," she said. "He says he'll hurt me if he catches me telling anyone."

The operator kept trying to get more solid information. The girl continued to refuse.

"I have three younger sisters," the girl confessed toward the end of the conversation. "Now, my daddy's having sex with two of them."

Finally, the operator convinced the girl that she would only be safe if someone from Liberty Godparent Ministries could get there to help her. At 2:00 A.M. the girl's line went dead again. By 8:30 A.M. that next morning the operator had notified our director who called a social service agency in Detroit. Before noon the director of that agency called Jim Savley with the full story.

"The girl's story is a nightmare," the social worker reported. "Her mother is completely paralyzed and totally helpless. The little girls, ranging in age from eight to fourteen, have been trying to nurse their mother without any outside help for more than three years. When we entered the house, the father was still drunk and asleep on the sofa. He was holding the twelve-year-old girl in his arms even as he slept. The mother's bedclothes had not been changed in days. There were more than twenty cats on the premises. The smell of human and animal excrement was overwhelming. The fourteen year old is in our clinic being tested for venereal disease. She is pregnant. The two other girls show definite signs of sexual molestation. All four girls, even the eight year old, show signs of physical abuse."

JoAnn had seen our toll-free number on a television ad for the Liberty Godparent Home program. She asked the social worker in Detroit if she could come to Lynchburg and talk about her unborn baby with "that nice lady on the phone." Within twenty-four hours JoAnn had been signed over to our custody by her father, and a Liberty University student who was returning to school drove her to 520 Eldon, where she stayed for five months.

Our director, Jim Savley, wrote letters to the court asking that the state step in and protect JoAnn and her sisters. He recommended that JoAnn's mother be sent to a nursing home, her father be prosecuted for child abuse and molestation, and the children be sent to foster homes.

It is our policy that a girl, no matter how young, be encouraged to postpone her decision about keeping the baby until the eighth month of pregnancy.

"We want her to deal with the reality of that living child," Jim Savley explains. "We want her to feel the movement of her unborn baby, to really know that a person is growing within her."

Even a fourteen year old like JoAnn has fantasized about getting married and having a baby. As she plays with her childhood dolls she is picturing them as living children. She escapes the horror of her own home life by dreaming of that day when she will have a home of her own. She escapes the reality of her cruel and drunken father by dreaming of the good and kind man she will marry. She escapes the reality of her own paralyzed and helpless mother by dreaming of the mother she will be to that imaginary little child of her own.

Then, suddenly, all of those long-visualized dreams to be a mother and have a baby are accelerated by an unwanted, unplanned pregnancy. She finds herself in a dorm room at our home surrounded by those same dolls of her childhood, but now there is a real baby kicking inside her. She has no husband and no home. But she wants that baby to love as she has not been loved. She is only fourteen years old. She is a victim of child abuse and sexual molestation. She is frightened, lonely, and without caring parents or any long-term friends. Yet, JoAnn must wrestle with issues most of us will never have to face.

I've walked through those dorm wings as a guest of the young women and the staff. I've sat and listened to them in the dining room or in the lounge as they struggle with the questions of adoption. I've talked and prayed and worried with them in the home, sitting beneath the great oaks or walking together over the grounds as they work through their feelings to make a final decision. Imagine the questions that JoAnn and the other young women like her must face.

If I keep the baby, how can I support it? How can I go back to school and finish my education? Will boys want to date me if I already have a baby? Will people make fun of me for being unmarried and having a child? Will it hurt my baby's chances by being illegitimate? Will my baby grow up without a father? What will the courts decide about my father? If they send me back to him, will he beat the baby or will he like the baby and quit beating me and my sisters because there is a baby in the house again?

If I place my baby for adoption, will it have a good home? Will I miss the baby terribly or will I be happy knowing a wonderful, Christian couple have the baby they've been praying for? If I gave my baby up for adoption would I be free to date, to fall in love, to get married, to have another baby, and start a real family of my own? Or would I feel so guilty about giving up my baby that I would never really be happy again? Will my baby hate me for giving him or her up or try to find me later on when he or she grows older?

Counselors from our Phase Three adoption agencies never force an unwed mother to make a decision against her will. If you are considering the founding of a Phase Three adoption agency in your community (and we hope you are) you must remember that a Liberty Godparent Ministries adoption agency is not profitable. We have not organized the agency for the primary purpose of placing babies into worthy Christian homes. Our first goal is to save the nation's unborn children by giving unwed young mothers like JoAnn the right to choose.

The difference between a Liberty Godparent Ministries adoption agency and a typical adoption agency is this: we are seeking the best possible Christian home for each baby entrusted to us for adoption. We are not seeking babies for worthy families waiting in the wings. That takes the pressure off us and off the young women we serve. We are free to help each young woman, like JoAnn, make her decision freely and with the highest possible degree of participation.

Of course each case is different. And each caseworker has his or her own professional bias. In JoAnn's case it seemed obvious that the best possible choice for her would be to relinquish her baby. JoAnn needed to be adopted or at least be placed in a foster home. Yet the courts in her state continued to ignore the situation. Nothing was done to help her or her sisters or her mother. How could she care for a newborn infant especially if she were forced to return to the nightmare from which she had just escaped?

Unfortunately, the younger and more naive unwed mothers are more likely to consider keeping their babies than older ones who are more realistic about the responsibilities of single parenting. JoAnn's counselor, her big sister, and the houseparents all stayed close to JoAnn as she wrestled with her decision.

Other girls who had given up their babies for adoption shared their experiences with JoAnn. We introduced her to adoptive parents who explained how they felt about their new babies. We showed her the papers she would sign and walked her carefully through each step of the adoption process.

JoAnn was fifteen years old the day her baby was born. She chose to keep her baby. Two weeks later, JoAnn's father persuaded his daughter to return to their hometown, where she could be near her family. "You don't have to live with us," he said.

JoAnn had changed radically during her time at Liberty Godparent Home. She had hoped to begin life on her own with her new seven pound, red-haired child. Our staff and many of JoAnn's new friends from LGH joined together that last day in the chapel of 520 Eldon Street to dedicate that beautiful new baby girl and her frightened young mother to God and to his safekeeping. We prayed that JoAnn would be strong enough to ignore her father's pleas to return to his house. A Christian woman in Detroit had opened her home to JoAnn and offered to help her with the baby.

It would have been easier to tell one of the overwhelming majority of success stories we have had through the services of the maternity and shepherding homes and adoption agencies, but this story raises all the difficult questions about abortion that you may be asking. Wouldn't it have been better for JoAnn to have an abortion in the first place? Shouldn't she have been the exception? She was a victim of incest. She was a child molested and made pregnant by her father. And worse, she was returning to her hometown, her life made even more complicated by a tiny infant daughter of her own. How long would it be before the baby was a victim, too? Was she already a victim?

I selected JoAnn's story because struggling with her kind of complex and confounding reality is the responsibility of any person who takes a serious stand against abortion. Talking about the issue is not enough. The lives of millions of young women and their unborn babies are at stake. They are not statistics to us in this ministry. They have names, faces, distinct personalities, and *worth*. Some of the women come to us from mansions, but most come from ordinary houses, and trailers, and tenements. Some were made pregnant by lovers and sweethearts. Most got pregnant simply by careless, irresponsible sex. Some were victims of incest or molestation. Whatever the origins of each pregnancy, there is a living child involved whose life hangs in the balance.

At Liberty Godparent Ministries we become entwined in people's lives. We share their suffering, and feel their pain. We prefer the stories of victory where young women are renewed by new hope and by new faith. In most cases the program works magnificently, but we do not ignore the unhappy endings. Whether the mothers we serve keep their babies or place them for adoption, almost without exception, they look back at the months with our staff and volunteers as a time when they experienced God's love in practical, helpful ways, perhaps for the very first time in their lives.

During her months at LGH, JoAnn felt God's love daily in ways she had never known before. She experienced a new kind of love from that awful moment when she called the crisis line and found a friendly, helpful voice to that moment at 520 Eldon when we dedicated JoAnn and her new baby into God's care. Who can measure the difference that experiencing real love has made on JoAnn's life or the life of her baby?

Our follow-up on JoAnn continues. She calls or writes us regularly, and recently she told us, "I am moving back with my father and sisters. If I'm there, I can make sure my dad doesn't mistreat my sisters....My family needs me to help take care of my mother, who is still at home." Since JoAnn is back in the terrible situation she left only a year ago, we pray together as a church and as a staff that God will reach out and help her deal with this situation—or perform a miracle in the life of her father. And we will always be ready to lend a helping hand if JoAnn again wishes to leave her home.

JoAnn called us because she wanted to save her baby. It was her decision. She was not forced or coerced in any way to make it. Perhaps our television special, "A Better Way," or our operators or our counselors influenced her decision against abortion. Our critics might feel that JoAnn's baby would be better dead than alive. We feel that is a harsh alternative, adding another evil to the evil already shaping JoAnn's young life. We are glad her baby lives.

JoAnn's story isn't over yet. We don't know what God has in mind for her little girl. Whatever it is, we are glad and grateful that God will have His chance in her life. It is risky business reaching out to people in despair. It is risky business helping babies be born into our world. We make plenty of mistakes along the way, but when given the choice of life or death for an unborn baby, we vote for life!

9
The Gift of the Shepherds

JENNIFER

I stood at my dorm room window, looking down at the long driveway leading to 520 Eldon Street. Missy knelt on the floor in front of me. Her face was pressed so close to the window that her breath was steaming up the cold glass window panes. She had smeared two damp eye holes on the foggy surface and was staring through them at the beat-up station wagon and the young couple that was climbing out of it. Kaye and Leona stood on either side of me, both so pregnant that they could hardly get close enough to the window to focus on the scene below.

"Quit steaming up the window, Missy," Leona complained. "I can see her but I can't see him."

"He's taken anyway," Gail muttered from her position at the second window in my room.

"She's so pretty," Missy added in a tiny voice below me.

"They look real nice," Kaye added. "You're lucky, Jennifer. I bet you're going to like living with them."

At least four or five other girls from the maternity home and our house mother, Mrs. Cook, were crowded into my room that day to watch the arrival of Linnie and Debbie

Dickson. They were coming to take me to their home, which they had volunteered as a shepherding home. I felt sad and excited at the same time.

Suddenly, "Big Mama" Leona put her heavy arm around my shoulders and whispered loudly, "We'll miss you, Jennifer. We'll miss you bad."

I picked up my suitcase and headed down the line of pregnant girls waiting to say good-bye. It was a wall of bulging bellies, tearful hugs and kisses, and quick words of endearment. Missy hugged me last. She had signed the final papers just that day to surrender all her maternal rights to the young couple that was adopting her baby girl. She would never see her daughter again. The gloom I was feeling was chased away by laughter as the entire dorm emptied noisily down the stairs, through the entry hall and out onto the driveway where the Dicksons were waiting.

Linnie Dickson was thirty-one years old. He was tall and curly headed and kind of country-looking. When he saw that moving mountain of pregnant girls come bursting through the door and down the driveway in his direction, he looked stunned and stood leaning on the door of his handsome but dented wooden-sided station wagon, staring at us with a cute but unsteady grin.

Debbie, his wife, was twenty-eight years old and apparently a real powerhouse. She was a social worker, the mother of two young children, a volunteer at their tiny Temple Baptist Church in Amherst, Virginia, and a devoted homemaker. She and Linnie—an interior designer—were remodeling their 200-year-old mansion in their spare time.

The Dicksons had volunteered their extra rooms to the shepherding home program, not because they needed something extra to do, but because they really believed in the program. Already, Andrea, a recent LGH "graduate,"

and her newborn son, Brian, were living with the Dicksons.
I would be their second live-in. Jim Savley was really high
on the Dickson family, but their home life sounded like a
zoo to me. Debbie walked right into that crazy crowd of
pregnant girls, grabbed my suitcase, and steered me toward
the car.

"Hi, I'm Debbie," she said smiling at me, "and that is Linnie." By then Linnie had recovered enough to take my hanging bag from Leona and my makeup kit from Kaye and to
begin loading them into the back of their wagon.

"Bye, Jennifer," Missy said as Linnie helped me into the
second seat. "Bye, Jennifer," the crowd of girls chimed in.

The engine coughed once ominously, then turned over.
Linnie steered through the crowd and away from 520 Eldon
Street. I looked back one last time at the girls already rushing out of the cold autumn winds back into the warmth of
their home away from home. Leona and Kaye were standing
arm in arm, still waving furiously at me. Missy stood alone
under the great oak tree, which was already leafless and
gray. Its giant branches were gnarled and moving slowly in
the wind. The tree looked like a huge, faithful watchdog
standing guard over Missy and my other friends as I drove
away.

"Mommy, tell Joshua to quit leaning on me," a voice beside me cried. I was not alone in that tattered wagon seat.
Eight-year-old Linnie was pushing his four-year-old brother,
Joshua, in my direction. Joshua was swaying back and forth
like a drunken sailor. They had interrupted Joshua's afternoon nap for the thirty-mile drive from Amherst to Lynchburg. He was too polite to fall asleep on a stranger's shoulder but his brother, Linnie, or "Scooter" as everyone called
him, was pushing him in my direction.

"Come on, Joshua," I said pulling that tousled head

gently toward me. "There's room for two in my lap." As he toppled into my arms half asleep already, he noticed the slight bulge where my baby was growing and carefully angled his weight onto my right leg.

"You gonna have a baby?" he said staring up at me through heavy lids.

"Yes," I answered. "One of these days."

"Good," he said grinning, then rolled over and fell fast asleep. Soon, both boys were sleeping. Linnie and Debbie and I whispered all the way to Amherst.

Scooter was Debbie's adopted son from an earlier marriage, and Joshua was Linnie and Debbie's foster son. Since Debbie was unable to give birth to babies of her own, she and Linnie planned to adopt other children. Someday children would fill that rundown mansion they were rebuilding in a country town in the Blue Ridge Mountains of Virginia.

"You'll love our house," Debbie said, leaning over the front seat and stroking little Joshua's curly hair as she whispered. "It's an old colonial straight out of *Gone with the Wind*," she added. "There are white columns on a magnificent veranda and a great oak door."

"I've been stripping old paint off that door for the past three weeks," Linnie added groaning. "Debbie won't be satisfied until we layer back two hundred years."

The Dicksons knew what I was feeling. They didn't push me to share. They didn't grill me about my "condition." They didn't judge or preach or advise. They weren't substitute parents. They weren't there to take care of me. They were providing a place where I could be pregnant in private. They were against abortion and wanted to do their part in saving babies' lives. To the Dicksons the issue was simple. What was growing inside me was not a mistake. It was a miracle. Abortion was wrong and someone had to help provide an alternative. They didn't have much, but what they had they volunteered.

"There it is," Linnie exclaimed proudly as we drove up the long, tree-lined driveway to their southern mansion.

"Looks like Andrea and Brian have come to welcome you," Debbie added.

A tall, rather pretty girl was standing on the porch surrounded by stacks of lumber and sacks of cement. She was holding her three-month-old son, Brian, cradled tightly in both arms. I could tell by the way she looked at me that Andrea knew exactly what was going on in my mind. She, too, had come to Lynchburg to have her baby. She, too, had moved into a stranger's shepherding home, wondering what would happen to her there.

"Hi," Andrea said as I climbed awkwardly from the wagon. "I'm Andrea and this is Brian." She whispered confidentially, "You're going to like it here."

I loaded my arms with bags and suitcases and followed Andrea into that huge old house. A hand-carved mahogany staircase curved away from the entry hall up to the floors above. The stairs were covered elegantly by a worn but still beautiful Oriental carpet. There was a cushion-covered windowseat halfway up the staircase, framed by a leaded bay window, looking down on the gardens below and at the distant, rolling hills.

"It's so beautiful," I said, looking about like a tourist, wondering if I would ever find my way around the place without a guide.

"I love sitting there when it's raining," Andrea said pointing to the windows and the view of the gray and cloudy sky.

Five huge bedrooms with twelve-foot ceilings were on

the second floor. The girls at LGH could have all been housed in the mansion with room to spare. My bedroom was all nooks and crannies and gingerbread trim. There were bookshelves built into the wall near the bed and old-fashioned closets that were so big they had dressers built right into them and light switches on the inside wall. Copper heating pipes connected all the rooms of the house, including the old servants' quarters and the huge covered porch down below, in a kind of primitive intercom system. On cold winter mornings the air would whistle through those pipes with a hollow, haunting sound like a freight train passing.

"Brr," I shivered, entering my bedroom on the second floor. "It's cold in here."

"It's cold everywhere," Andrea answered, draping a down quilt over my head like a tent. "Pretend you're camping," she added, rolling her eyes.

The ancient coal furnace built to heat the mansion didn't work. No heating company could coax it back to life. There were fireplaces in the bedrooms, but most of them didn't work either. On cold Virginia mornings the wood-burning stove in the main sitting room drew us all together from our frozen little outposts about the house. I soon learned to stay downstairs near that glowing stove until it was time for bed and then race upstairs and jump beneath my downy quilts, preserving all the body heat I could to get me through the night.

I kept a bottle of distilled water in my room to clean my contacts before and after wearing them. After one very cold winter night, I found the bottle of water frozen solid. But there were plenty of quilts and padded jackets and a constant, blazing fire in the fireplace in the living room and in the sitting room stove. And there were plenty of chores to keep our bodies busy and our minds distracted from the cold.

The last four months of my pregnancy went by quickly. I shared all the housework with Debbie. She let me practice my underdeveloped homemaking skills on our extended family. Almost every day we filled the house with the aroma of freshly baked breads and cakes, newly ground coffee, soups and stews and casseroles.

There were trips into town for counseling, group therapy, and prenatal classes. I used every possible excuse to return to 520 Eldon Street for seminars or just to see my friends. And though I attended church with Linnie and Debbie in Amherst, we often went together to the meetings at the Thomas Road Baptist Church in Lynchburg.

J. J. Yelvington, my social worker from Eldon Street, visited every two weeks and kept a careful journal of my physical and mental health. My folks wrote almost every day and called several times a week to see how I was doing. Kaye called occasionally, and even Missy sent a card now and then from her home in Florida.

Debbie insisted that I attend the Lamaze natural birth classes at the local Virginia Baptist Hospital. These classes trained the husband and the wife to handle each stage of the unborn baby's development up through and including the actual delivery. The husband would be present almost as midwife. That meant I would need a partner in the classes and Debbie Dickson volunteered.

"I can't do it," I said to Debbie as we mounted the stairs to the hospital seminar room to attend the first Lamaze class.

"Why not?" Debbie asked, turning to face me on the stairway.

I didn't answer.

"Of course," she groaned, hitting her forehead with the palm of one hand. "I'm sorry," she added. "Sometimes I am so dense."

She grabbed my hand and pulled me up the stairs and into the women's room outside the seminar classroom.

"What are you doing?" I asked, as Debbie stood at the sink soaping her ring finger and pulling at her wedding ring.

"I'm finding out how fat I've gotten since my wedding day," she answered laughing. Then she handed me her ring.

I took it in my hands and stared at her. I almost cried.

"Cut it out," she said. "We'll both be crying. Put it on. Nobody will ever know."

After class we joined our fellow students for a pizza at Amherst's only pizzeria. Two of the couples were members of Thomas Road Baptist Church. They talked to Debbie about volunteering their homes to Liberty Godparent Ministries after their own babies were born. Because I was the youngest member of the class, they made me class mascot. They accepted and loved me. I never needed to wear Debbie's ring again. But that one time sealed our friendship forever.

Each night after the Lamaze class Debbie and I sat up late reading the chart and reviewing the pictures of the child developing inside me. I learned the baby could already hear and recognize my voice. He curled, stretched, sucked his thumb, and squirmed for his favorite comfortable position to sleep, just as I did at night in my bed in that cold mansion. The more we read, the more we marveled at God's creative genius.

"What do you mean the baby decides when to be born?" I asked Debbie late one Tuesday evening. When I was first pregnant, I resented the notion that some little person was imposing on my body, making it grow, making me feel sick, giving me stretch marks, disrupting my life. Little by little I grew to love and respect the child growing inside me and to congratulate myself for the part I played in his development. It tickled me to think my baby would make his own decision to be born, when he felt ready. I smiled when I thought about it. He was stubborn, just like his mom.

"The baby decides when she wants to be born," Debbie said again. She always called my baby "she." And I always called him "he." I don't know why. We both refused to call him "it." "The books says so, right here," Debbie added defensively. "One day," she read, "your baby will know it is time to be born. That decision is your baby's and your baby's alone."

After those late-night sessions with Debbie, I wanted to keep my child more than any time before or after. But I knew with equal certainty that my baby needed a father and a home and a family. I admit that occasionally I had a fantasy that Jeff would grow lonely and restless without me. On a few winter nights, when I huddled alone in that great cold bed, I sometimes pictured Jeff driving from Macon to find me and take me home again. But in the warmth and light of morning I knew he wasn't ready for marriage or for the responsibilities of being a husband, let alone a father. I had to be content to have this fantasy warm me on those cold and lonely nights in Amherst.

Little Brian was a real comfort during those times. Early in the morning, while the house was dark and the moon was still high overhead, Andrea would slip little Brian into bed with me on her way to work the breakfast shift at a restaurant on the highway just outside of Amherst.

"Good morning, Brian," I would say, awakening to find him sleeping soundly beside me.

Andrea's baby slept on his back with one arm folded across his red "Tough Guy" pajama top and the other arm bent so his thumb could be firmly planted in his mouth. He grinned and grimaced as he slept. I wondered what dreams he might be having as I leaned on one arm, looked down at his little face, and thought about the baby sleeping inside of me. I wondered if my own little baby could be dreaming about that day when he would decide to leave the safety of his amniotic sac and come kicking and screaming into this world. I wondered what his future would be. I wondered if I could give him up to that future and trust him into God's care. I had decided from the beginning to surrender my child for adoption, but the closer the day came, the more complex that decision became.

"I couldn't do it," Andrea told me one afternoon. "I planned to offer my baby for adoption," she said, "but when the moment came to leave the hospital without him, I couldn't do it."

We were sitting on the windowseat on the landing above the garden. The first snow of winter had fallen, outlining branches of the trees in a sparkling white. The morning sun reflected off that icy world and made rainbow fragments in the leaded glass.

"I had signed the first papers," she told me. "A young couple had been notified. But when the time came, I couldn't let him go."

Andrea couldn't return home to North Carolina. She had become a Christian at the Thomas Road Baptist Church. Her father was a violent, unforgiving man. Her mother was dead. Her boyfriend was a small-time drug dealer who wouldn't like the changes in Andrea's life-style. She was afraid to go back home. She had to forget her past and start a new life with Brian in Virginia. Debbie and Linnie had taken her in through the shepherding program until Andrea could build a new life for herself and for her baby. She had found a job. She was searching for an apartment. It had been a difficult decision but every day Andrea felt more confident she had made the right choice for them both.

"What about you, Jennifer?" Andrea asked me that day as we watched the icicles dripping down the windowpane.

"I'm going to give my baby up for adoption," I said, "if I can follow through on it."

Andrea didn't say much more. She just took my hand and stared silently at the endless white outside our window.

That next morning I called Dr. Morrison at the Liberty Godparent Ministries offices in Lynchburg. He was the director of child adoption services and the gentlest man I've ever known. I scheduled an appointment to begin the actual adoption process.

"Are you sure, Jennifer?" he asked me. "Take all the time you need."

I looked down at my huge swollen abdomen. I felt as big as the side of Linnie's barn. My greatest fear, those awful stretch marks, had become a distinct reality. I thought I was seven months pregnant, but I was really late in my eighth month.

"I'm ready now," I answered.

Dr. Morrison made it perfectly clear that I could help shape the future for my child. Although I would never know the adoptive parents by name, I was to be included in their selection. I wanted my son to grow up in a loving, Christian home where he could experience the love I had known in my own home and with the Dickson family. I told him that I hoped he would select a couple that couldn't have children of their own because that would help me feel that I was doing something even more special in letting my baby live. Dr. Morrison used to fuss and fidget if I was even five minutes late for those adoption counseling sessions. He was afraid I would slip and fall in the snow or that Debbie's car would run off the road. He always jumped up from his desk and ran around to greet me smiling broadly and gesturing for me to be seated. Every visit we talked about my baby and his future and what I dreamed for him.

Then one afternoon just before Christmas the discussion took a new direction.

"We've a young couple," he said, "that seems perfect for your baby."

I was stunned. It was really happening. Someone out there was being prepared to receive my baby. They didn't know who I was or when my baby would be born. The LGH program refuses to take away the mother's option to keep the baby up to the very last moment. But as Dr. Morrison described the couple to me, I felt more and more excited about my baby's future with them. At the same time I felt more and more afraid that I could not give him away. I kept wavering back and forth, even though my increasing size told me I would have to make a decision very soon.

Despite my vow to stay as close as possible to my normal size, I had gained thirty-five pounds. Because of my size, life became miserable. I waddled when I walked. Joshua watched me sitting down on the living-room sofa one day and said, "Look, Mommy, Jennifer sits down in pieces." He was right. I didn't sit, I lowered my body, section by section. The house didn't seem cold anymore. Even breathing made me sweat. I was fat and tense and uncomfortable most of the time. The days dragged by slowly. Finally, it was Christmas Eve.

"Help us with the tree, Jennifer," Scooter said, climbing up a ladder to place a silver star at the top of a beautiful pine Christmas tree that almost filled the mansion's living room.

While I napped, the Dicksons had raised the tallest Christmas tree I'd ever seen in a home. The ceiling was thirty feet high in the entry hall near the stairway and the tree reached almost to the ceiling. Already it was loaded with sparkling colored bulbs and golden balls reflecting the light. Christmas gifts were stacked under the tree. The smell of evergreen and candles and Christmas candies filled the room.

"Hi, Jennifer," a familiar voice said from somewhere in the living room.

"Daddy!" I screamed and waddled quickly down the stairway. My father took me in his arms. Mom was close behind. We cried and laughed and held each other beneath the Christmas tree.

"Surprise!" said Linnie bashfully.

"Surprise!" Joshua and Scooter joined in.

"Surprise?" I said. "It's a dream come true."

During the visit Mom and Debbie spent most of their time together in the warm kitchen. Dad and Linnie toured the house and grounds, talking wood and paint and shingles.

When I wandered into the kitchen the next morning, Mother was making my favorite cinnamon rolls. I knew that I was too fat to eat them, but the fragrance of the fresh dough and the melted butter and sugar and cinnamon drew me to that room like a magnet. As we talked, the three of us took turns thumping the bread dough and watching it rise again.

"We certainly appreciate your taking Jennifer in like this," my mother said. I noticed that her lip trembled and she looked embarrassed as she spoke.

Debbie noticed too. She looked at my mother closely and then sat down beside her.

"Mrs. Simpson," she said, "you don't think for a moment that Jennifer is here because you or your husband failed in some way, do you?"

Mom looked surprised. Her eyes filled with tears.

Debbie dried her hands on a clean dish towel and leaned against the kitchen table.

"Jennifer is in this shepherding home for many reasons," Debbie said quietly, "but none of them should make you feel one bit guilty."

"We should have kept her at home," my mother blurted out. "We shouldn't have sent her away."

It was the first time I realized how deeply hurt my mother felt about my time in Lynchburg. She thought that she had failed. Debbie quickly set her straight.

"Liberty Godparent Home is not a place that just babysits pregnant girls because their families don't know what to do with them," Debbie began. "The prenatal care and instruction that Jennifer has been getting here would not be offered in most communities."

Debbie leaned forward as she talked. "If Jennifer had stayed at home, she would have had no other young women to share the experience. Here she has friends, counselors, dorm parents, people who are trained and people who really care."

I watched my mother begin to listen. Debbie was not about to let this moment slide.

"It is not a shameful thing to be in a shepherding home. You know how the public feels. You know how innocent, well-meaning friends can make a mess of things. Jennifer needed a safe, private place to save her baby. Staying at home could have complicated the process and endangered the baby."

Suddenly, Debbie's tone changed. She took my mother's hands and said quietly, "I suppose the best reason to explain why Jennifer is here is this: We want her here. It gives us a chance to be a part of the wonderful thing she is doing."

"Thank you, Debbie," my mother said. "You will never know how much those words mean to me."

That Christmas Eve dinner provided a memory that will never fade. We sat at one long table, Debbie and Linnie Dickson, Scooter and Joshua. Andrea and her little baby, Brian, were there, and Mom and Dad and me, looking something like Mary must have looked that Christmas Eve two thousand years ago. Before dinner, eight-year-old Scooter read the Christmas story from the Dickson family Bible. He faltered on some of the words and read very slowly, but the familiar story never sounded more beautiful to me.

" 'For there is born to you this day in the city of David a Savior, who is Christ the Lord. And this shall be a sign to you: You will find a Babe wrapped in swaddling clothes, lying in a manger.' And suddenly there was with the angel a multitude of the heavenly host praising God and saying 'Glory to God in the highest, and on earth peace, good will toward men!' "

When Scooter finished reading, Linnie asked Dad if he would pray the Christmas prayer. His eyes brimmed with tears as he stood and looked down the long table. First he smiled at me. Then he smiled at Mom and the Dicksons, Andrea and the children. I was afraid he couldn't speak. Slowly he bowed his head and began to pray.

"Oh, Lord," he said, "thank you for this family, for this food, and for Christmas." He paused and swallowed hard. "Because of this wonderful day none of us will ever be the same."

"Amen," said Scooter Dickson, grateful for a short prayer and a very big turkey.

"Amen," I added as Daddy squeezed my hand beneath the table and winked at me through grateful tears.

10

Will You Save a Baby?

JERRY

On New Year's Eve in 1984, fifteen minutes past midnight, as the sounds of bells and sirens and "Auld Lang Syne" were dying away, a tremendous explosion ripped through the Hillcrest Women's Surgical Center in Washington, D.C. The abortion clinic there was damaged extensively. The blast was so powerful it broke more than two hundred windows in apartments and offices across the street. Agents from the Federal Bureau of Alcohol, Tobacco, and Firearms, together with District police and the F.B.I., carefully combed through the burned and blackened ruins. A task force of federal, state, and local officials launched a nationwide manhunt for the abortion clinic bomber. It was the thirtieth attack on an abortion clinic since 1982, the fourth attack in the same week.

Through the press coverage of the violent and inappropriate series of abortion clinic bombings, the nation was reminded again that since *Roe* v. *Wade* more than a fourth of all pregnancies in our nation end in abortion. The estimated sixteen million babies who have died since the Supreme Court's decision represent four thousand abortions every day. In some states, like New York, the number of abortions has been almost as high as the number of live births. The nation has gradually wakened to the terrible reality that an entire generation of unborn babies is in danger.

Slowly the national debate grew in intensity. Men and women who had never been politically active took to the streets to protest abortion. Grandmothers and young children marched side-by-side carrying placards and wearing protest pins. A steady stream of anti-abortion letters and telegrams poured into the offices of national, state, and local officials. Although it was tragic and wrong that abortion clinics were being bombed or vandalized, a *Newsweek* editor wrote that the bombings were further proof that "the national debate over abortion has reached literally explosive levels."

Unfortunately, some men and women in the media accused me and the Moral Majority of encouraging, if not initiating, these violent acts. It wasn't true. I am glad to share the credit of mobilizing millions of people to take a peaceful stand against abortion. I am glad that their united voices are being heard and are making a difference. I am glad that millions of young women facing unwanted pregnancies are thinking twice before they agree to having their babies killed. But I am not glad when anyone stoops to violence, and I am just plain angry when the media accuse me of participating in any way in those violent acts.

It is not the first time I have been falsely accused of being an advocate of violence. In 1981, Bartlett Giamatti, president of Yale University, warned his entering freshmen class that I "have licensed a new meanness of spirit in the land, a resurgent bigotry that manifests itself in racist and discriminatory postures, in threats of political retaliation, in injunctions to censorship, in acts of violence."

Portions of his speech blasting me and the Moral Majority were used on the front page of the *New York Times* and in pages of *Time* and *Newsweek* magazines. This is only a small sampling of the millions of words printed and spoken against me in the past ten years in newspapers and newsmagazines, on radio and television, in sermons and speeches, in political cartoons, satirical musical reviews, on bumper stickers, and even on obscene greeting cards.

Of course there are times when I am tempted to defend myself against the charges that they invent against me. Of course there are times when I feel angry and hurt and misunderstood. But the greater the lies against me, the more certain I am of eventual victory. The question is no longer, "Are we going to win the fight against abortion?" Now it is merely a matter of "When?"

Just days after that terrible bombing in Washington, D.C., my wife Macel and I were standing beneath the Capitol rotunda at President Reagan's second inauguration. Millions of dollars had been spent to celebrate this historic event with parades and festivities on the streets and in the beautiful parks and monuments of our nation's capital. Tens of thousands of celebrants had traveled to Washington, D.C., to join in the celebration. But the weather was too cold. Since the wind-chill factor was forty-two degrees below zero, the extensive outdoor inaugural festivities were canceled by the president, and the swearing-in ceremonies were held inside the Capitol. Only two thousand of us could fit beneath the great Capitol dome. My wife and I stood with Mrs. George Bush and the vice-president's family as President Reagan delivered his second inaugural address.

He spoke frankly and eloquently that day of the dignity and worth of human life, and of his own position against abortion and the deaths of unborn children. Later I learned that sources close to the president had advised him to delete this controversial material, but he had refused. Now, during the first year of his second term, he has instructed the attorney general to begin a dialogue with the Supreme Court that could eventually strike down *Roe* v. *Wade* and end this decade of death.

The day following the inauguration I joined 72,000 people who braved the icy temperatures to march down Pennsylvania Avenue to the steps of the Supreme Court for the twelfth "March for Life," coordinated by Nellie Gray and pro-life groups from across the nation. The president's voice echoed out across that vast sea of faces, applauding our stand against abortion and encouraging us to continue fighting for the rights of unborn children until we finally secure their right to life. As I stood to address that huge crowd of people shivering in the capital's cold winter chill, I knew we could win the battle.

Yes, we can win the fight against abortion without taking to the streets in real warfare, without bloodshed, without bombing abortion clinics or abortionists' offices, without acts of violence and hatred. Using the rights granted us in a democratic system we can judicially and compassionately turn our free society from its killing course and become a model for the rest of the world for the right to life of every child, born or unborn.

As I looked down across that great crowd of pro-life friends, I thought about the price they and their organizations have paid to save the lives of our nation's unborn children.

I knew it hadn't been easy for the Moral Majority (or for any of us associated with it) during those first years. The press had ridiculed us. The pornographers smeared and satirized us in their magazines. Liberal politicians remained aloof. Many elected officials didn't even bother to return our calls or respond to our letters or petitions. Bumper stickers appeared saying: "The Moral Majority is neither." Political cartoonists portrayed me as a Hitler figure and warned America that I was out to destroy the democratic process and to force my brand of Christian faith on everyone else. Our meetings were picketed, often by sincere people who believed the lies about us. Our lives and our families' lives were threatened.

We learned quickly the price that must be paid for taking a stand on the issues of importance to us. We are Republicans and Democrats and Independents. We make mistakes, and when we do, we seek forgiveness. We are new on the political scene and we are learning the art of influencing government. In spite of the fury of the opposition, of our own occasional ignorance and naivete, of our own exhaustion and fears, of the silliness and the slander hurled against us, we continue to have faith in our nation and in its political system. Already in these few short years, we are making a difference.

At this moment there are more than 6.5 million active volunteers working under the banner of the Moral Majority. Our *Moral Majority Report* newspaper is mailed to more than one million homes a month, helping voters understand the issues without political rhetoric and gobbledygook.

We have hundreds of thousands of volunteers (which included 102,000 pastors during the 1984 election) helping in voter registration. In the past six years we've registered over eight million new voters. In one day, after carefully examining the goals of our organization, 569 preachers from the Ministerial Alliance of one major American city joined the Moral Majority en masse.

We've helped elect congressmen and senators who support our goals, and we've helped to unseat some of the most powerful men in government who opposed those goals. We've convinced thousands of major retail stores to remove pornography from their shelves. We've worked hard for stronger legislation combatting drug traffic and enforcing penalties against the people who supply drugs to our children. We've launched an extensive, nationwide program of education on the major issues facing our country, especially the abortion issue. And our education program against abortion, along with other fine pro-life programs around the country, is having a real effect.

Last year, for the first time since the Court's decision in 1973, the number of abortions actually went down in our country. And we've helped elect a president who has promised, if given the opportunity, to help create a Supreme Court that will reverse the tragic decision to legalize abortion and help stop the killing.

But a victory against abortion is not enough. We need to work just as hard for the health and happiness of the girls and women who are facing unwanted pregnancies and for the future of their babies after they are born. That introduces Phase Four of our dream.

As I write these words early in September 1985, there are already two hundred Phase One Liberty Godparent Ministries across the nation. We need a total of ten thousand to meet the coming demand. That means there are only 9,800 groups to go. In Phase Four we plan to mobilize this force of volunteers. Will you be one of them? Let me explain how.

You might want to initiate a Phase One program in your community. Remember, Phase One is a completely volunteer operation that almost any person or church, service club or charity, can develop. Our national offices will provide all the help you need to begin a Pregnancy Crisis Center in your town. We will help you train volunteers who will operate your local crisis hot line for the young girls and women in your community who have absolutely no one else to talk with about their fears concerning an unwanted pregnancy. We will help you give free pregnancy tests and show you how to counsel or mobilize volunteer counselors for the women who call. We will help you launch your first shepherding home and organize volunteers to teach your girls during their long months of pregnancy the important life skills or crafts they will need or enjoy in the future. Also we will provide materials and practical "know-how" for a complete community awareness program about abortion and "a better way."

There are approximately fifty Phase Two LGH programs already in action around the nation. These programs include everything described in Phase One plus a residential care facility or group maternity home for underaged women who need a place to live during their months of pregnancy. We have a carefully detailed manual to assist you step-by-step in starting a Liberty Godparent Home. We hope you will visit our home in Lynchburg or another one nearer you to talk to the staff and volunteers and to see how they set up their home. Then call our toll-free line to find out how we can help you do it too.

We hope to have ten thousand shepherding and maternity homes across the nation. If each Godparent Center helps 150 girls and women a year, that means 1.5 million young women will have experienced "a better way." At no cost to the woman or the taxpayer, the lives of 1.5 million babies will be saved every year.

If the current number of abortions continues to decline, at least 750,000 more babies will be available for adoption every year. Remember, last year's estimates range from two million to five million homes that were qualified for adoption with only fifty thousand babies available. Imagine the disappointment. Imagine the loss. There are loving homes waiting for every child we can save.

Finally, during the next few years, we will need hundreds of Phase Three adoption agencies to place the tens of thousands of newborn children with their waiting families.

Chances are right now in your town, in your neighborhood, even on your street there is a young woman who faces an unwanted pregnancy. Picture her. She may be the girl who checks your groceries after school or sells you Girl Scout cookies. She may be the pastor's daughter or the mayor's niece. She could be any one of the attractive young women you see in church, entering the schoolyard, or babysitting your own young children.

She is not an evil person. She just made a simple mistake. In an unguarded moment she let her need for intimacy get the best of her good sense. Now, a living being is growing inside her. She is only a teenager but suddenly she must make a difficult decision about the life or the death of her unborn baby.

When she finally has the courage to tell someone, she will almost invariably be advised to get an abortion. "It is only a fetus", they will tell her. "It is not human. It will feel no pain. The whole thing will be over in a few minutes. It is harmless and it won't cost you anything."

Well-meaning family and friends, counselors, teachers, and pastors have been spreading that falsehood for years, but we know the truth, and we must tell it. We are tired of doctors and parents and friends, even pastors and teachers of this nation's young people, pretending that a fetus is only unthinking, unfeeling tissue when in fact it is a human being waiting to be born. We are tired of the abortionists' lies about the "painless" effects of abortion on the unborn child and the "harmless" effects of abortion on the unwed mother.

Let's face it, this cycle of misinformation has led to the use of abortion as a primary birth control technique. Our kids are ignorant about sex. According to competent research, American teens commonly believe that pregnancy cannot result from the first sexual intercourse. Nevertheless it can and often does. It happened to Jennifer. Too many teenagers also believe pregnancy cannot occur if sex occurs infrequently. In fact, one moment of sexual intimacy between a teenage boy and a teenage girl is all that is required to create a brand new living soul. Recent surveys of America's young people found that there is even a common misunderstanding that if they have sexual intercourse in a nonhorizontal position, that conception is impossible. Biologically any method of sexual intercourse can lead to conception, and ignorance, half truths, and lies only lead to increasing the difficult and dangerous problems we are facing.

Since 1972, the number of teenagers who are sexually active has risen by two-thirds. Today 49 percent of all fifteen to nineteen-year-olds are sexually active, according to the Guttmacher Institute. It reports that the average teenager today starts sexual activity at age sixteen and that half of teen pregnancies occur within six months thereafter. Last year, guided by the misinformation provided them by their parents, their friends, their doctors, and even their churches, more than half a million of those teenagers tossed down their money for a "quick and easy" abortion to solve the problem of an unwanted pregnancy.

We believe that if teenagers are old enough to be sexually active, they are old enough to be informed clearly of the consequences of those actions. The long term results of the current lies about abortion are becoming more and more apparent. Believing the lies, a teenager gets an abortion, returns to her home or classroom, and eventually discovers the truth about the effects of abortion on the fetus and upon herself.

From that moment at least one common behavioral pattern is all too clear. The young woman may feel anger at those who encouraged her to abort her baby. She perceives them as having betrayed her by holding back the long-term truth for the short-term solution. She may feel more and more depressed and humiliated as she realizes the implications of what she has done. Many young women carry the emotional and physical scars of an abortion with them forever. Or worse, as the number of teenage abortions increases, so does the number of teenage suicides by girls who cannot live with the growing guilt and grief they feel.

Right now a girl on your street, in your neighborhood, or town may be lying alone in her room or walking in a park or sitting in a library or coffee shop, desperate and afraid, praying for someone to help her. Picture the hundreds of thousands of young women right this moment who are in that predicament. Let me tell you the story of one girl whom I know. Then, Jennifer will finish her story and you will be left with an important decision.

Gail was standing on the wing of a 747 jetliner at a gate in Chicago's O'Hare Field when they found her. No one knows exactly how she got there. She was crying "bitterly," the police report reads. "Her arms were reaching to heaven and her body was twisting and turning as if in terrible agony. She had torn off her clothing and stood on that giant wing as nude as she was born." Airport security personnel got Gail down from the wing and into a restraining area of the concourse before they questioned her. She had overdosed on an illegally manufactured "pleasure" drug. Since her arms were perforated by old needle marks, the authorities surmised she was addicted to heroin.

A social service agency got Gail into a drug rehabilitation program, where she dried out in three months and showed signs of being a rather normal, even intelligent, young woman. When she was discharged from the drug detoxification unit, she took a bus to the Liberty Godparent Home in Lynchburg.

"I came to save my baby," she told our director, Jim Savley, when he began the intake interview. "I saw the movie on TV about what you do here and I came to give it a try." Jim Savley will never forget what happened next.

"After her first night in the maternity home," Jim recalls clearly, "a nurse brought Gail into my office at exactly 10:00 A.M. We had not admitted her officially or selected the shepherding home that would best minister to her needs."

Jim Savley is a seasoned cop, a social worker, a pastor, and the chief administrator of Liberty Godparent Ministries.

He has seen all kinds of girls enroll. But he is still surprised occasionally by the variety of deep personal needs he discovers in each young woman who comes our way for help.

Jim selected Gail's shepherding home with great care. The couple who volunteered their home was given careful training. Gail was assigned daily meetings with a trained, professional counselor and was also assigned a mature big sister who could be her friend and monitor along the way.

"Not every story has a happy ending," Jim reminds us. "But Gail's story is an accurate testimonial to what happens to most of the girls and women who go through the Liberty Godparent Ministries program."

"On a Wednesday night," Jim reports, "four months after Gail moved into the shepherding home, she and her big sister were attending a Bible study-prayer meeting at Thomas Road Baptist Church. Gail was about to have her baby, and all through the meeting she had sat crying quietly and wiping away the tears. During the benediction she turned to her friend and whispered loudly, "I want to become a Christian before my baby is born."

Her big sister grabbed Gail's hand. They hurried from the meeting into the old sanctuary, now a chapel and a quiet place of prayer where they sat down in the last row of pews and began to talk about the Christian faith.

"I've really messed up," Gail said. "Do you think God can forgive me?"

For the first time in her four months at the Liberty Godparent Home she told her own horror story in complete detail. Having run away from home at thirteen, she found work in the city as a prostitute, smoking an occasional marijuana joint, then snorting cocaine, and finally mainlining heroin. Her heroin habit was costing Gail four hundred dollars a day when she climbed out on that airplane wing in desperation. She was selling her body day and night to pay her drug addiction bills. She was afraid that no one could ever really forgive her, not even God.

Gail's big sister opened her Bible to John 8:3–12 and told the history of a young woman who was thrown at Jesus' feet by an accusing mob. She read Jesus' own words to those who could not forgive.

"He who is without sin among you, let him throw a stone at her first."

She also read Jesus' words to the adulteress after the humbled mob had stolen quietly away leaving the woman alone with Jesus.

"Has no one condemned you?" He had asked.

"No one, Lord," she answered, looking around in surprise and disbelief.

"Neither do I condemn you," Jesus said. "Go and sin no more."

Gail sat quietly. The words of promise shattered the fear and the guilt she had carried since she was thirteen years old. Then she began to pray. That night, Gail experienced the same love and forgiveness in her life that another young adulteress had experienced two thousand years before.

Several days later, Gail's baby was born. She offered the child for adoption through the Liberty Godparent Ministries agency, asking that her child be adopted into a family that didn't live near a city with dark, lonely streets like the ones she had known. Today, Gail is working in a suburban town, almost a village, in Tennessee. She is a Sunday school teacher in a country Baptist church. She visits Lynchburg on those Memorial Day celebrations at the Liberty Godparent Home in May. Her life was changed because she decided to save her baby. And Gail's story is just one of hundreds we could tell.

There is another side of the story that must be told. Jennifer and I have been sharing stories of the young girls and women who are pregnant and need help in saving their unborn children. But what about the boys and men who make these women pregnant? What happens to them?

Needless to say there are many horror stories of incest, and of rape, and irresponsibility, but there are also new data coming out of our informal follow-up studies of many of the fathers of the children born to mothers in the program. It is good news. We think it should be told.

Gary is seventeen. He is a high school junior who fell madly in love with a sophomore girl in his hometown. They had courted seriously for a year without any sexual involvement until after an out-of-town football game, when they were invited to a private home where marijuana was the main attraction. Neither Gary nor his young friend was experienced enough to handle the passions that followed. Four months later Judy, Gary's girlfriend, was admitted to our home in Lynchburg.

At this point most people assume that Gary would just disappear, as Jeffrey had disappeared from Jennifer's life. It is an assumption by most of us that the young men involved in most of these unwanted pregnancies are irresponsible and uncaring. However, more and more we are learning that many of the fathers, especially the teenage fathers, are as loving and responsible as any married father might be.

With the support of their parents for whatever decision they chose to make, Gary and Judy decided they were too young to get married and that they should put their child up for adoption. While Judy was with us at 520 Eldon Street,

Gary wrote and phoned regularly. He sent gifts and flowers to Judy and encouraged her during those long months away from home. After the baby was delivered and Judy had recuperated sufficiently to return to her home and family, Gary appeared with Judy's mom and dad to take her home.

It's important not to rely on false assumptions that all men are irresponsible and uncaring. Some of the young women we assist find that the young men who made them pregnant want to help care for them during their pregnancies. We have strict rules against dating during a girl's time at the maternity home. But we have found that some of the young fathers like Gary will understand and abide by the rules, at the same time doing everything possible to share the responsibility of the pregnancy in every way that they can.

There are still young men who advise their girlfriends to get an abortion or who walk away from any responsibility for what has happened. They, too, made a moral decision to have sex without a marriage commitment. They, too, have created a human being. And they, too, are responsible for this human being's life or death.

Since January 1982 the program has worked with more than twenty thousand pregnant girls. Out of all those cases, 99 percent have chosen against abortion to save their unborn babies. And none of the young women who have entered our maternity homes has ever opted for another abortion. The Liberty Godparent Homes are making a difference.

Will you seriously consider joining us in helping save the unborn babies in our nation? Will you think about the possibilities of volunteering to help establish a Liberty Godparent program in your town or neighborhood?

There are people who smile when they hear my dream. Of course it is too large to accomplish. Of course it can't be done in a few short years. Of course it will require tens of thousands of volunteers, tons of materials, millions of hours spent in training and preparation, and thousands of dollars for satellites to handle millions of calls to crisis hot line centers across the nation. It will necessitate tens of thousands of shepherding homes, thousands of maternity homes, and hundreds of adoption agencies. But we can do it! We must do it! And we will alter the course of history if we try to do it!

11
Honk and Wave Backward

JENNIFER

The wipers on Andrea's yellow Datsun hatchback strained against the little snow drifts forming on her windshield. The back wheels spun on the icy surface as we slid into the last open place in the lower parking lot of the Thomas Road Baptist Church.

"We did it," Andrea gasped as she switched off the ignition and turned to lift her baby, Brian, from his car seat in back.

"But why?" I groaned from the passenger side where I had been wedged between the seat and the dashboard for the thirty-mile skid from Amherst to Lynchburg. "Why didn't you let me and Brian off up there by the church and park the car on your own?"

Andrea was grinning to herself and pushing Brian's arms into his quilted snowsuit.

"You could have parked near a bus stop or taxi zone," I complained. "You could have rolled me out the door as we went by and I could have bounced into the sanctuary without losing a moment."

Andrea laughed out loud. Brian looked at his mom and turned to share her smile with me.

"You keep out of this, kid," I threatened. "Your mother is trying to kill me off just before I have my baby."

"Shut up and start walking," Andrea said with a grin and a prod. "You are getting too fat. You need the exercise. Hold on to the rail. You'll be fine."

There was a large crowd of church members waiting to cross at Thomas Road. One of the young husbands from my Lamaze class waved and shouted, "When are you going to have that baby, Jennifer?"

"I've got another month to go," I called back.

Twenty people turned in my direction smiling sympathetically. Just that moment the blue stretch van with the LGH girls drove by and honked, a tradition when passing other LGH girls on the street. When the van driver honked madly, the girls in the van would turn and wave in the wrong direction, and the girls on the street, co-conspirators in the tradition, would also turn their backs on the van and wave in an equally wrong direction. Then, watching the confused looks on the pedestrians' faces, everyone would dissolve in laughter.

That morning we played the usual greeting game, and I'm afraid the little crowd from Thomas Road Baptist Church is still wondering if the home is for the mentally ill.

Mr. and Mrs. Cook were waiting at the church entrance to greet us.

"Looks like little Stephen will be worshiping with us next Sunday," Mrs. Cook announced prophetically. "You'd better not get too far from home this week," she added with a knowing whisper as we walked up the aisle toward our front row seats.

I had chosen Stephen for my baby's name. I was convinced I was going to have a boy after Dr. Falwell had preached on Stephen, the first Christian martyr. Stephen would be courageous and strong and faithful like his name-sake.

The church was crowded. There were more than two dozen girls from LGH sitting in our front right section. At first I had been embarrassed to join them in "fat city." We were all so obviously pregnant and husbandless and away from home. But the people at Thomas Road loved us. They smiled and waved and hugged us when we arrived and when we left the sanctuary. They invited us out for rides or meals. They provided us clothing and gifts and special treats. They dedicated our babies into God's care and keeping, and many of them promised to pray for us and for our babies daily. The program itself was their finest gift to us. Through their support and that of the television viewers of "The Old-Time Gospel Hour," we had a place to save our babies. They were proud of us and what we were doing.

I sat on the front row that day because I couldn't wedge comfortably between the pews. I loved those informal moments before the service began when Macel Falwell, Dr. Falwell's wife, played the grand piano. There was a great pipe organ as well, and many Sunday mornings a full symphony orchestra joined in from the left balcony. Television cameras were wheeled into place as the choir moved slowly onto the platform. Special guests sang and played, and the congregation joined in the singing. Then as Dr. Falwell stood in the pulpit to read his text from the large Bible, I opened my Bible and got out my yellow marker pen to underline and make notes as he preached.

My life had changed during those months in Lynchburg. God became real to me there, more real than He had ever been before. I felt His love in that place through these people in ways I had never felt it. That morning as I looked up

at the great white pulpit I began to cry quiet tears of gratitude. I would miss this place. I would miss these people.
Even as I prayed, I felt Stephen begin to stir. Maybe he heard
the grand piano and the orchestra playing. Maybe he heard
the choir singing:
"Great is Thy faithfulness, Oh, God my Father.
There is no shadow of turning with Thee.
Thou changest not. Thy compassions they fail not.
As Thou hast been, Thou forever wilt be."
Stephen jumped and kicked inside me throughout that
entire service. I could almost hear him singing. I think he
heard the music that morning and decided it was time to be
born. Thank God he waited twelve hours more before he
acted on his plan.

At 5:30 A.M. Monday morning I awakened. I had spent the
night with Andrea in her new apartment in a small town between Amherst and Lynchburg, because I just didn't want to
drive the extra miles to the Dickson's place.

I groaned loudly. Andrea rushed into the living room and
found me sitting straight up on the couch with my feet on
the floor, rubbing my stomach, and looking dazed.

"Are you OK, Jennifer?" she asked peering into the darkness of the room.

I sat without moving. Stephen was moving enough for
both of us.

"I think I'm going to have a baby," I finally answered. "But
there's no sure sign yet," I added. Although the Lamaze
classes had us totally prepared for this moment, I felt afraid.
It was good to have Andrea there.

"Call me at work if you need me," she said heading out
the door. "And don't worry. People have babies every day."

She kissed me on the forehead. I looked at Brian all bundled up against the cold to go to the babysitter's.

"See you tonight, kid," I said to him. "You might just have a playmate to come home to."

The door opened and closed. They were gone. Now I wished I were in that giant old shepherding house in Amherst where Debbie and Linnie, Joshua and Scooter, were sleeping. I was alone. Andrea would not reach work for another twenty minutes. Suddenly, I felt a desperate need to get to the bathroom and knew the moment had come to announce my news to the world.

I called the Dicksons, even though they were thirty miles away. "I'm having a baby!" I yelled into the telephone.

"Wonderful," Debbie yelled back.

"It's about time," I heard Linnie muttering sleepily in the background.

"Wonderful?" I gasped back at Debbie. "I'm going into labor and I'm all alone and you're a billion miles from here and…"

"Get a grip on yourself," Debbie ordered. "You know that there is plenty of time after your water breaks to get you to the hospital. Get ready. I'll be there in thirty minutes. Linnie will call Dr. Callister. He'll meet us at the hospital. You know the plan."

She was calm. I was panicked. I could hear Joshua and Scooter cheering in the background. "Jennifer's going to have her baby," Scooter shouted. "Yippee!" Joshua answered back.

The moment I hung up the phone, I decided I didn't want to go through with the plan, not any of it. I didn't want to go to the hospital. I didn't want to start labor. I didn't want to have a baby. I was scared. But we were family. Debbie and Linnie would come through for me. Andrea would be by my side. Jim Savley, the Cooks, Dr. Morrison, all the girls would be outside my window cheering. I had left my home in fear, and in Lynchburg I had found a second loving family. And they would see me through it.

But I was still scared. Those next twenty-nine minutes were excruciatingly long. Debbie Dickson arrived ahead of schedule. Labor had just begun. She shoved me lovingly into the back seat of that battered old station wagon and began the drive to the Virginia Baptist Hospital in Lynchburg.

"Sorry," she said each time she hit a bump in the road.

"Forget the bumps," I groaned in reply. "Just get there quick."

I tottered into the hospital's emergency entrance while Debbie parked the wagon. I filled out the entry forms. They wheeled me into the elevator and down the long tan corridor to the maternity ward. Debbie caught up with me. She looked at her watch and waited for me to announce the next short, quick cramp.

"They're ten minutes apart," she said as I was being settled into the labor room. "Should I call your mom?" Debbie asked quietly.

"Yes," I answered, "but tell them not to come. I'll call them the minute Stephen is born."

The pains were coming harder and quicker. I tried to see it objectively. Women have been having babies since the beginning of time, I tried to tell myself. Thousands of women across the world were having babies at that very same moment, I reasoned. But all I could think about was the pain. I grabbed the sides of that hard bed and hung on tight. My knuckles were white. I groaned and moaned without caring who heard me.

"Debbie," I yelled, "where's Debbie?"

"I'm right here," she said, hurrying into the room. "I had to sign some admission papers."

"I'm dying," I complained, "and you're off signing papers."

Debbie stood beside me and rubbed my back and whispered words of encouragement. I yelled and groaned and called her names. It was not my proudest moment.

"Breathe," Debbie said, "just like we learned at class."

The pain was terrible. I took it out on Debbie. She never lost her patience. She never turned away. She just rubbed my back and whispered quietly, "Breathe, just like in class."

"What do you know," I finally yelled at her. "You've never had a baby."

She grabbed my hand and held it tight. I looked at her and wished with all my heart those words had not been spoken. She forgave me with a wink. I rolled my eyes and shook my head in embarrassment. She just laughed.

"I'm dying," I said. "I can't do this. I want to quit!"

"You're doing great!" she said. "It'll be over in no time."

The nurses were watching my progress.

"She's dilated about eight centimeters," I heard one say. "Call Dr. Callister."

Moments later I was in the delivery room. Hands were lifting me and rolling me onto the delivery table. Lights shone brightly overhead. Dr. Callister's sparkling blue eyes and neat gray hair appeared upside down above me. From behind his green paper mask I heard him asking questions and giving orders. Debbie never left my side. She held my hand and guided every breath. I was gasping to her count, crying short, painful sobs, and pressing down as the doctor ordered.

"It's a boy," Debbie whispered at the end of interminable pain. I opened one eye and then the other. Dr. Callister's eyes were scrunched up with pleasure. He was holding Stephen in his hands. Stephen looked mad.

"So it wasn't easy for you either," I whispered.

I lay there on my back looking up at him. He was red and terribly small and more beautiful than anything I had ever seen. As I looked at him, I realized the pain had ended. I didn't hurt anymore. I remembered a verse Debbie had read once from the Gospel of John.

A woman, when she is in labor, has sorrow because her hour has come; but as soon as she has given birth to the child, she no longer remembers the anguish, for joy that a human being has been born into the world.

Already, the pain was forgotten. A child had been delivered into the world and I had done it. The tears streamed down my temples and into my ears. Debbie stood beside me crying and squeezing my hand and telling me she loved me. The nurses were grinning. They knew all the time how it would end. And Dr. Callister paraded about the delivery room holding Stephen proudly for the world to see.

"Dad," I practically shouted into the phone in the recovery room, "you have a healthy six pound eleven ounce baby grandson."

"His name is Stephen Layne," I shouted to my mother. "He's beautiful."

Dad gasped and his voice got thick. Mom laughed with delight. I talked endlessly of my labor and delivery, but especially of my beautiful baby son. In the middle of a sentence I remembered. He was my son, but only for a while. Soon, Stephen would belong to someone else. I couldn't talk anymore. Debbie hung up the phone. For a moment I stared at her. I swallowed hard and tried not to cry. She didn't move. Suddenly, she was holding me and both of us were crying.

"How can I give up my baby?" I said between the tears. "How can I give Stephen away?"

Debbie had never known the joy I felt that day, but she had known that sorrow. We comforted each other. Debbie prayed a loving, quiet prayer for God's presence in our lives. I dozed and woke throughout the rest of the day. Each time I awakened Debbie was sitting there in the room beside me. At about 4:00 P.M. a nurse arrived, carrying my son wrapped in a light blue blanket.

"Time to feed your baby," she said placing Stephen in my arms. She bent over, smelling of White Shoulders perfume, and told me how to support his head and how to feed him without getting bubbles of air into his stomach. Then she and Debbie left Stephen and me alone. I held my baby and wanted to hold him forever. There were things I wanted to say, things I knew he would not understand or remember.

They had wrapped Stephen in a little flannel receiving blanket. I wanted to unwrap him and look at every part: the shoulders, the knees, the toes, the little reminder of his previous life still embedded in his tummy. He had long skinny fingers, just like mine, and the same pointed chin that I remembered from my own baby pictures. I stared at him. I didn't know I could ever love anything as much as I loved my son Stephen that day he was born.

"Do you know that I love you, son?" I whispered into his

tiny ear. "Will you remember? We have to trust God now. He'll take care of you. Will you forgive me? Will you love me anyway?"

Words poured out of me. Stephen looked as if he was trying hard to understand. Maybe one day, when he reads these words, he'll know how much I love him still.

When they took him back to the nursery, I pulled the thin yellow blanket up so that the nylon edge was touching my face. The heavy drapes covered the huge windows. It was twilight outside. The room was almost dark. I was alone again.

Twenty-four hours later a nurse wheeled me through those long hospital corridors. Debbie walked beside me carrying a bouquet of flowers that had just arrived. Linnie was parked on the street. Joshua and Scooter came running to greet me. My arms were empty, so I could hug the children.

"You had a baby?" Joshua asked as we drove back to the old mansion in Amherst.

"I had a baby," I answered, trying desperately not to show him the terrible grief I carried.

"Was it a boy?" little Joshua asked innocently.

"Yes, it was boy," I answered.

"And somebody will adopt him?" Joshua wondered. "Like mom and dad adopted me?"

"Oh yes, Joshua," I cried picking him up in my arms and holding him tight. "Just like your mom and dad adopted you."

We rode the rest of the way home in silence. I knew in my heart that I had made the right decision. Still I carried an overload of grief and guilt. It was Joshua who comforted me the most. I pictured Stephen in his place. I pictured the young girl who gave up Joshua feeling as terrible as I felt. If only I could tell her about Debbie and Linnie Dickson. If only I could sit with her in the window box in the wonderful old mansion in Amherst and show her Scooter and Joshua at play. If only she had known and loved that family as I had known and loved them, she would not worry or feel guilt or grief any longer. She would know that God can be trusted to care for His little children.

By Friday Mom and Dad had arrived to take me home. Linnie Dickson carried my suitcases to my dad's car. Debbie and Mom chatted on the porch. I knelt by the tree swing and talked to Joshua and Scooter one last time. Andrea and Brian surprised us with one last noontime visit. Then everybody hugged and cried and waved good-bye. I stared out the back window of our car until the old mansion and my second loving family disappeared in the distance. At Lynchburg there were papers to sign and more hugs and tears and waves good-bye. Then we were on the highway home.

Years later, I returned to Lynchburg as a student at Liberty University, another ministry of Dr. Falwell's Thomas Road Baptist Church. In my dorm room there is a tiny Polaroid snapshot of Stephen in the delivery room. In the envelope with that photo is a letter to my baby that I wrote before he was born. It was a class assignment at LGH. I didn't know then the pain I would feel for his life after meeting the Dicksons. I often read the letter when I feel sad and I am thinking about Stephen in the arms of his new mom and dad. Although many months have passed, there isn't much I'd want to change.

If I Should Die Before I Wake

Dear Stephen,

I think the most important thing for you to know is that you were not unwanted. Many, many people care for you and pray for you, but none more than me. I want the very best for you, and if I could give it to you, don't think for a moment that I wouldn't.

God has a very special plan for your life and right now it's for you to have both a mother and a father.

Not a day in your life will go by without your being in my thoughts and my prayers. And even more important than that, God has His eye on you.

Never once since that instant you were conceived has God taken His eye off you, and not until the moment you cease to exist will He. I pray that you will grow and mature in the knowledge that God gave up His son, Jesus Christ, who sacrificed His precious life for you and me.

This love and concern for you exceeds even mine. I love you.

Your mom,

Jennifer Simpson

12
A Day of Celebration

JERRY

The magnificent old house at 520 Eldon Street was ablaze with balloons, banners, and bunting. A band was playing in a red, white, and blue gazebo erected temporarily near the trailers that served as classrooms. A huge "A Day to Remember" sign was draped between the second floor windows of the dormitory wing. Hundreds of folding chairs were being set in neat rows on the freshly cut lawns. Microphones had been tested and speakers set in place. Parked cars filled the long curving driveway and all the streets for blocks around the Liberty Godparent Home in Lynchburg, Virginia. Volunteers were directing traffic. People carrying picnic baskets were squealing with delight at the first sight of old friends. Visitors were rushing across the grounds to hug and kiss and reminisce. Babies were everywhere.

"Dr. Falwell!" I heard the voice before I saw Missy running toward me, her arms filled with programs and her pockets full of granola bars. "Take one," she said, holding up the colorful outline of the Memorial Day celebration. "We're having a party."

She hugged me awkwardly. Programs spilled onto the grass. As I stooped to help her gather up the programs, I looked into her face and knew what the Liberty Godparent Ministries was all about. A huge smile had replaced the tense, drawn look.

"Thanks," she said, backing away, her arms filled with programs again. "Thanks for everything."

She didn't need words to make herself perfectly clear that day. Missy had arrived at 520 Eldon only thirteen years old and five months pregnant. She was only fifteen that afternoon in May, yet Missy had experienced more grief in her few years than most adults experience in a lifetime. An abused and sexually molested child made pregnant by a "friend of the family," Missy came to save her baby, even though she had wanted to die. Instead of death she found new life on Eldon Street. Her baby boy had been adopted by a wonderful Christian doctor and his wife. Missy had finished junior high and was doing well as a high school sophomore. She was a new person with many wonderful memories of this place, and she had returned to celebrate those memories with dozens of girls whose stories were not unlike her own.

As I walked amid the festive decorations, I could feel the intense love the young women and their families had for this place and for each other. One by one they approached me to thank me for what the people of Thomas Road Baptist Church and volunteers and supporters from across the nation had done to save their lives and the lives of their babies.

"Look, Mommy," I overheard a little boy cry out, "somebody's dead."

The child was staring at the small marble memorial we

had moved into place for that day of memorial and celebration. That single stone stood in memory of the sixteen million babies who had been aborted since the Supreme Court's *Roe* v. *Wade* decision in 1973. His mother knelt beside the stone and began to explain why it had been placed there. She promised to show him the larger stone, dedicated to unborn children in the beautiful grotto on the campus of Liberty University. She spoke quietly for just a few moments. Then he took her hand and they walked together toward a small group of friends.

I watched them join the others and knew what that young mother was probably thinking but couldn't say about the tombstone. "There but for the grace of God go you, my son." She was one of the first young mothers admitted to the Liberty Godparent Home. He was one of the first babies we had saved.

On Memorial Day, the last Monday in May, while the nation remembers the brave young men and women who have died on battlefields across the world, we remember the unborn children who have died from abortion. Of course we are grateful for those who have died defending our nation during the wars of these last two centuries, and we remember and honor the 116,516 American men and women who died in the First World War, the 405,399 Americans who died fighting in World War II, the 54,246 more of our young people who died in Korea, and at least 56,000 who died in Vietnam. In those seventy-two years more than 600,000 American men and women have died in those four bloody wars, but in the last twelve years at the very least sixteen million American babies have been killed by abortion. For every one American killed in warfare in this century, twenty-five babies have been killed in their mother's womb in the past twelve short years. Who will remember them if we don't?

"Dr. Falwell?" Standing beside me at that tiny memorial was Andrea, Jennifer's friend and former roommate in the Dickson's shepherding home in Amherst. She was holding her baby son, Brian.

"Andrea, you look wonderful," I answered. "And your son is getting so big."

"I'm thinking of entering him in the Ten-Yard Toddle this year," she said grinning. "Do you think it's too early for his first gold medal?"

We walked slowly toward the Memorial Day baby games. Volunteers were lining up each event. Babies and young children were being prepared for the Five-Yard Crawl and the Mom-Baby Relay. Hundreds of spectators were gathering. In that crowd were adoptive parents, mothers from LGH, and newlywed graduates of the program returned to show off their new husbands and families. Of course, there were babies of every size, shape, and color. There were also volunteers and their families from Thomas Road Baptist Church and from the other churches around Lynchburg who help Liberty Godparent Ministries.

"Hold Brian a minute, will you?" Andrea asked suddenly. "I haven't signed up for his entry number."

She raced away from me toward the entry area. I looked down at the beautiful baby in my arms. He was almost eight months old. His eyes searched my faced uneasily at first, for his mother had suddenly disappeared into the crowd leaving him in the arms of a stranger. He puckered up to cry.

"Don't cry, Brian," I urged softly. "Your mommy's coming right back." I could see Andrea in line with other mothers across the grass. "See, she's right over there," I added.

Brian slowly relaxed but he continued to stare at me. His eyes sparkled. His cheeks were red. He looked healthy and happy and loved.

"He's a cutie, isn't he?" Andrea said, once she returned with baby Brian's Five-Yard Crawl entry number.

"Yes," I answered as I held him up to get his number pinned to the back of his summer jumpsuit with the special knee pads.

"Padded knees?" I said curiously. "Is that common?"

Andrea winked at me. "We're going to win this event," she said. "We've been training."

Andrea had carefully sewn little pieces of padding from an old football uniform into the knees of Brian's jumpsuit. She took him gently from me and began to coach him for his big event.

"Don't look back," she told her infant son. "Just get out there and crawl like mad."

Brian smiled at his mother and reached up to touch her face, not understanding a word of it. Andrea didn't mind. She hurried to get her young champion into place.

Babies were being placed on the grass behind a white-ribbon starting line. The finish line was placed exactly five yards away. Tension began to mount. Dads and moms, grandpas and grandmas, staff and volunteers, visitors and special guests crowded the infield. People buzzed with excitement. Judges took their places. The starter raised his flag. Mothers put their babies on the line.

"On your mark!"

"You can do it, Brian," Andrea whispered loudly from the sidelines.

"Get set!"

Already babies were crawling about, milling back and

forth across the starting line. People were beginning to cheer. The babies were bumping into each other and rolling over on the lawn, laughing and playing with the starting ribbon.

"Go!"

"Come here, Brian," yelled Scooter Dickson from his place near the finish line just a few feet away. "Look what Uncle Scooter has for you."

Brian loved Joshua and Scooter Dickson. And the huge red balloon that Scooter was carrying was a clear and wonderful target. Brian began to crawl toward Scooter. Andrea began to cheer. Jennifer Simpson and the Dicksons crowded around the red balloon, urging Brian on.

Five feet. Four feet. Three feet. Two feet. The balloon was one foot away. Brian had the gold medal by a twelve-inch crawl. At that very moment, Scooter accidentally let go of the balloon and it soared into the oak tree overhead. Its string tangled in the branches. Brian stopped and looked up at the balloon.

"No, Brian," Andrea yelled.

"Crawl!" Scooter encouraged, motioning wildly.

"Go for it!" Debbie Dickson yelled.

The crowd went wild. Brian stared up at the balloon. Suddenly, he turned over on his back to get a better view of it hanging there. That's when Brian lost the race. I thought the people in the cheering section would strangle on their laughter as they watched that wonderful child, perfectly content, pointing at the balloon and smiling. His mother rushed to Brian when the other children had all crawled by. She cradled him in her arms and smiled as friends and family crowded around to congratulate Brian on his near victory.

At the awards ceremony, every child was given a prize. I wandered from picnic table to picnic table, sampling the southern fried chicken and watermelon and listening to the stories that were being told. Tammy, the first young woman admitted to our Liberty Godparent Home, was eating with her mother and a group of girls from "the class of 82." Beside her sat a young man I didn't recognize.

"Dr. Falwell," she shouted when she saw me coming, "we're over here."

Tammy was almost eighteen years old that Memorial Day. Her handsome young son was three. Even as we talked, I felt a tug at my pant leg.

"This is Timothy," Tammy said.

I picked up her son and hugged him tightly.

"And this is his daddy, Carl." A tall, blond seminary student from Chicago came around the table to shake my hand.

"I don't agree with all your politics, Dr. Falwell," he said politely, "but you saved my son and I'll always love you for that." For a moment I stood looking at that proud and obviously intelligent young man. Then I patted him on the back.

Carl and Tammy had met at a Lutheran youth convention when Tammy was just fifteen. They were married a year after that and immediately Carl applied to adopt Timothy as his legal son and heir. Our political differences, whatever they might have been, seemed a million light years away that day as we sat and talked about the future of this beautiful family and the role that the program had played in their young lives.

At a nearby table I spotted Bonny and her parents who had come all the way from Shreveport, Louisiana. They had much news to report. Bonny's father was the preacher who had begged me to get Bonny into the program at a ministers' meeting two years before.

"We're all doing beautifully," Bonny's dad reported to me that day. "Look at us," he said. "We're a family again."

Gail, the girl who had once stood naked on the wing of a 747, had flown from Ohio to share her story. "I remember one special morning in chapel at 520," she said to a small group of friends who gathered around us. "I had a few demerits," she explained. The girls who knew her best laughed loudly.

"A few demerits?" one cut in sarcastically. "You had the limit."

"Remember the time you tried to climb in the van for the Wednesday night trip to Thomas Road Baptist wearing only red hot pants and a string top?" a third girl chimed in.

"Stop it," Gail ordered. "You're right. I had every demerit in the book and had invented a few on the side."

Gail smiled and looked away thoughtfully. Our little crowd of listeners grew quiet. They loved Gail, and they respected her. They had seen an incredible change in her life during those months at the Liberty Godparent Home and her return that day was proof that those changes would last.

Gail turned and looked at me.

"Dr. Falwell," she said quietly, "do you remember that time in chapel at 520 when you spoke on God's forgiveness?"

I couldn't remember, but I nodded anyway.

"At the end of his talk," Gail said turning to her friends, "Dr. Falwell announced that all our demerits were 'officially forgiven,' 'canceled,' he said, 'rubbed out.' As of that moment, he told us, 'we had a clean slate.' "

Suddenly, I remembered the chapel Gail was describing. The girls had cheered and applauded my announcement wildly. Gail was especially enthusiastic. Now I understood why.

"I asked you after chapel why you did that," she reminded me. "You told us that you wanted to show us in a practical way what God has done for each of us."

Gail's eyes filled with tears. "And for the first time I understood," she said. "I really was forgiven. I really could begin my life again."

In the shadow of the giant oak just outside her old room at LGH, Gail remembered the day she experienced God's forgiveness for the very first time. On this Memorial Day she was surrounded by her friends, girls who had experienced the same kind of love in that wonderful old mansion. As I walked away from that happy, celebrating crowd, they had their arms around each other and their faces were streaked with tears.

The band began to play a rousing patriotic tune as the chairs around the speaker's lectern filled up rapidly with the program's graduates, their friends, and families. I sat on the little makeshift wooden platform with Jennifer Simpson. Both of us had been invited to speak briefly about the program. After Jim Savley introduced the special guests, a children's choir stood to sing.

There must have been thirty-five or forty children in the group, ranging in age from six to ten years old. They were grubby from the games and stained with brownies and chocolate chip cookies and melted ice cream. They blinked against the bright sunlight as they filed quietly into place. The crowd grew silent as the children began to sing:

213

Jesus loves the little children;
All the children of the world.
Red and yellow, black and white,
They are precious in His sight.
Jesus loves the little children of the world.

As they sang, I looked out at the children gathered on the lawn. There were dozens of older children sitting in the shade of those great oak trees and there were infants wearing victory ribbons sleeping in their mother's arms, exhausted by the Five-Yard Crawl or the Mother-Baby Relay.

As I heard the children singing, it was easy to understand why God would love them. What was hard to imagine were the reasons why our nation still permitted the slaughter of millions of unborn children just like them every year.

I studied that faithful group of staff and volunteers sitting in the folding chairs or on blankets spread on the grass. They were doing something about the slaughter. At that very moment inside the house phones were ringing. As we sat listening to the music, crisis hot-line operators were at work talking to young women who had called wondering if we could help them save their babies. Those Godparent Center operators were fighting on the front lines of a battlefield that stretches out across the nation. Even while the children sang, the battle between life and death went on inside 520 Eldon Street.

From where I sat I could see pregnant girls standing at the open windows inside the old mansion, listening to the children singing. In their own personal battle between life and death, they had made the choice for life. We who support the work of saving a baby risk almost nothing for the children. Those pregnant teenage girls are risking everything to save their unborn babies. Each girl was alone in a city far from home. Each was frightened and ashamed. Each was struggling with the painful implications of the decision she was making about abortion and adoption. Each was worried about going home and starting life again.

I knew that one day soon those same girls watching from their windows would be with the crowd on a Memorial Day picnic. One day they would join Missy, Tammy, Gail, Leona, Kaye, Andrea, and the others in celebrating the lives of the children they had saved. One day they too would know for certain that their decision to save a baby had been the right decision. But as they stood looking down on us from their dormitory windows, that future day of celebration must have seemed a long way off.

The children finished singing and the audience applauded enthusiastically. Jim Savley stood to introduce a young graduate of the program who had volunteered to share her story with that crowd. It would take courage for Jennifer Simpson to speak. A sophomore at Liberty University, she was a good student and was planning a career in public speaking and broadcasting. She was looking forward to dating and marriage and raising a family of her own. Until that moment none of her present classmates knew about Jennifer's abortion or her second pregnancy. Only her roommates at the Liberty Godparent Home knew that she had spent six long months here and in one of our shepherding homes. No one even imagined the pain and the sorrow this beautiful young girl and her family had carried.

Jennifer walked quickly to the microphone. I could see her mom and dad sitting proudly in the very first row, looking up at their brave and beautiful daughter. Both parents were clutching handkerchiefs and smiling proudly as Jennifer stood to speak. Debbie and Linnie Dickson sat beside them with Joshua and Scooter. Leona and Kaye and

Missy smiled up at Jennifer, their eyes filled with tears. Missy waved. "Good luck," she whispered. Andrea sat on the grass just below us, holding little Brian fast asleep in her arms. He still wore his jumpsuit with the padded knees. Jennifer smiled and began to speak.

As she told her story, the same story that she has shared with you, I looked down at that little boy asleep in her friend Andrea's arms. Whenever I think of babies like Brian or Jennifer's son, Stephen, or of the hundreds of babies just like them that have been saved through our program and others like it, I think of what might have happened if people hadn't cared enough to save them. As I sat on the platform listening to Jennifer and watching Andrea's son, I imagined their children sliced into pieces and suctioned from their mother's womb or burned and blackened by salt poisoning and born dead. I thought of the seventeen thousand bodies of unborn babies discovered in one California dumpster and the bodies of thousands more being burned in a large Kansas City incinerator.

"You are alive, little Brian," I said quietly to myself. "Thank, God, Stephen, you are alive!"

Jennifer finished her story and sat down between her mother and her father. Mr. Simpson placed his arm around his daughter's shoulder and hugged her proudly. Jennifer's mother took her hand. Debbie and Linnie looked on tearfully. Leona and Kaye were smiling. Missy was leading the audience in their applause. Andrea leaned over and kissed her sleeping baby. I noticed that she had pinned to Brian's light blue jumpsuit the brightly colored ribbon from his near victory in the Five-Yard Crawl. The ribbon read, "A Day To Remember."

"They are alive," I said again to myself as I stood to speak. "What more is there to say?"

Notes

Chapter Two

1. Bob Woodward and Scott Armstrong, *The Brethren* (New York: Simon and Schuster, 1979), p. 238.

2. Ibid.

3. Ibid., p. 239.

4. Ibid., pp. 239–40.

5. Roe v. Wade, 410 US 113 (1973).

Chapter Four

1. *Our Throw Away Society* (Topeka: Right to Life of Kansas, Inc.). To obtain, write: Right to Life of Kansas, Inc., Crosby Place Mall, 717 So. Kansas Avenue, Topeka, Kansas, 66603.

2. Ibid.

3. Gary Bergel, *When You Were Formed in Secret* (Elyria: Intercessors of America, 1980), pp. 1–2.

4. *National Right to Life News,* Oct. 14, 1982.

5. Ibid.

6. Ibid.

7. Ibid.

8. Bergel, *When You Were Formed*, pp. 2–4.

9. Vincent J. Collins, M.D., Steven R. Zielinski, M.D., and Thomas J. Marzen, Esq., *Studies in Law and Medicine: Fetal Pain and Abortion—The Medical Evidence* (Chicago: Americans United for Life, Inc., 1984), preface.

10. "Church Homes Offer Alternatives to Abortion," *New York Times*, Jan. 31, 1984.

11. Collins, Zielinski, and Marzen.

12. John Lofton, "Unborn Suffering Is a Veritable Fact," *Washington Times*, Feb. 10, 1984.

13. Vincent Collins, *Principles of Anesthesiology*, 2d ed. (Philadelphia: Lea & Febiger, 1976).

14. John Lippis, *The Challenge to Be 'Pro-Life'* (Santa Barbara: Pro-Life Education, Inc., 1982), p. 9ff. Available through National Right to Life Educational Trust Fund, 419 7th Street, N.W., Suite 402, Washington, D.C., 20004.

15. Margaret Wynn and Arthur Wynn, *Some Consequences of Induced Abortion to Children Born Subsequently* (Collegeville, Minn.: Foundation for Education and Research in Childbearing, 1973).

16. Thomas Hilgers, M.D., *Induced Abortion, A Documented Report*, 1976.

17. G. Dixon and J. Richardson, "Letter: Effects of Legal Termination on Subsequent Pregnancy," *British Medical Journal*, 2 (July 31, 1976), 299.

18. F. Glenc, "Early and Late Complications after Therapeutic Abortions," *American Journal of Obstetricians and Gynecologists*, 1 (Jan. 1, 1974), 34–35.

19. F. Glenc, *American Journal of Obstetricians and Gynecologists*, 5 (1977), 556–9.

Notes

20. Lippis, *The Challenge,* p. 10.

21. J. Stallworthy et al., "Legal Abortion: A Critical Assessment of Its Risk," *Lancet,* 2 (Dec. 4, 1971), 1245–9.

22. John Willke, M.D., *Handbook on Abortion* (Cincinnatti: Hayes Publishing Co., 1979).

23. Lippis, *The Challenge,* p. 10.

24. Ibid., p. 11.

25. Milling, "The Men Who Wait," *Woman's Life,* Apr. 1975.

26. G. Dixon, J. Richardson.

27. Carl Tishler, Ph. D., "Adolescent Suicide Attempts Following Elective Abortion: A Special Case of Anniversary Reaction," *Pediatrics,* 1981, no. 5.

28. Lippis, *The Challenge,* p. 16.

29. Sheppard, *British Medical Journal,* 1 (1976), 1303–4.